THE PSYCHIATRIC INTERVIEW

THE PSYCHIATRIC INTERVIEW

Fourth Edition

Daniel J. Carlat, M.D.
Publisher
The Carlat Psychiatry Report
The Carlat Child Psychiatry Report
The Carlat Addiction Treatment Report
Associate Clinical Professor of Psychiatry
Tufts University School of Medicine
Boston, Massachusetts

Practical Guides in Psychiatry
Daniel J.Carlat, M.D.
Founding Editor

🌐 Wolters Kluwer

Philadelphia • Baltimore • New York • London
Buenos Aires • Hong Kong • Sydney • Tokyo

Acquisitions Editor: Jamie Elfrank
Product Development Editor: Andrea Vosburgh
Production Project Manager: Kim Cox
Design Coordinator: Stephen Druding
Manufacturing Coordinator: Beth Welsh
Marketing Manager: Rachel Mante Leung
Prepress Vendor: SPi Global

4th edition

Library of Congress Cataloging-in-Publication Data
  Names: Carlat, Daniel J., author.
  Title: The psychiatric interview / Daniel J. Carlat.
  Other titles: Practical guides in psychiatry.
  Description: Fourth edition. | Philadelphia : Wolters Kluwer, [2017] | Series: Practical guides in psychiatry | Includes bibliographical references and index.
  Identifiers: LCCN 2016008384 | ISBN 9781496327710
  Subjects: | MESH: Interview, Psychological—methods | Mental Disorders—diagnosis | Physician-Patient Relations | Handbooks
  Classification: LCC RC480.7 | NLM WM 34 | DDC 616.89/075—dc23 LC record available at http://lccn.loc.gov/2016008384

To my patients, past, present, and future. Thank you for allowing me to ask you question after question, and thank you for answering so honestly.

Foreword

The Psychiatric Interview is straightforward, practical, and wise, yet often lighthearted and funny, a breath of fresh air where comparable references have often been boring and ponderous. It brims with extraordinary gifts for its readers. It is a scholarly review of the research literature, yet it moves swiftly and has a light, even jaunty, tone. It is very much up-to-date and serves as a useful introduction to many ideas, such as those from psychodynamics, that are not widely available to contemporary students.

Best of all, the book is alive, an extraordinary achievement in view of the amount of detailed material presented. It emphasizes the *person within the patient* and the need to form an *alliance* with that person to secure reliable information and cooperation in treatment. We *feel* the patients presented by Dr. Carlat; they are not simply diagnoses. Dr. Carlat offsets the profession's reputation for being cheerless and pathology minded; he illustrates many ways by which effective relationships can be formed and shows how relationships that are endangered can be repaired, perhaps especially at the close of an interview.

The Psychiatric Interview is designed in an easily accessible format, with aids for memory, appendices for organizing information, and sensible guides for recordkeeping. This is teaching by example at its best, with the examples both vivid and pointed, so that they stick in the reader's mind.

Truly understanding another human being is a daunting challenge, yet nothing is more important if we are to soothe the suffering of a ravaged soul. Use this book as a guide to reach for that understanding.

Leston Havens, M.D.
Professor of Psychiatry, Emeritus
Harvard Medical School
The Cambridge Health Alliance
Cambridge, Massachusetts

Preface

Over the course of a 40-year professional career, you will do ~100,000 diagnostic interviews. The diagnostic interview is by far the most important tool in the arsenal of any clinician, and yet the average training program directs relatively few resources to specific training in the skills required for it. The general assumption seems to be that if you do enough interviews with different kinds of patients, you'll naturally pick up the required skills. That may be true, but it can take a long time, and the learning process can be painful.

I hatched the idea for this manual one night during my first year of psychiatric residency. Starting my shift in the acute psychiatry service (APS), I noticed five patients in the waiting room; the resident who handed me the emergency room beeper said that there were two more patients in the emergency room, both in restraints. At that moment, the beeper sounded, and I called the number. "Psychiatry? This is Ellison 6. We have a patient up here who says he's depressed and suicidal. Please come and evaluate, stat." That meant that I had a total of eight diagnostic assessments to do.

As the night stretched on, my interviews got briefer. The developmental history was the first to go, followed quickly by the formal mental status examination. This trimming process continued until, at 5 a.m., it reached its absurd, but inevitable, conclusion. My entire interview consisted of little more than the following question: "Are you suicidal?"

As I handed the beeper off to my colleague at 8 a.m. (I had slept for 50 minutes, about the length of a psychotherapeutic hour), I began to think about those interviews. Were they too short? (I was sure they were.) Were they efficient? (I doubted it.) Had anyone come up with a system for conducting diagnostic assessments that were rapid but at the same time thorough enough to do justice to the patient?

Looking for such a system became my little project over the rest of my residency. I labeled a manila file folder *interviewing pearls* and started throwing in bits and pieces of information from various sources, including interviewing textbooks, lectures in our Wednesday seminars, and conversations with my supervisors and with other residents. When I became chief resident of the inpatient unit, I videotaped case conferences and took notes on effective interviewing techniques. Later, during my first job as an attending psychiatrist, I practiced and fine-tuned these techniques with inpatients at Anna Jaques Hospital and outpatients at Harris Street Associates.

What I ended up with was a compendium of tips and pearls that will help make your diagnostic interviews more efficient and, I hope, more fun. Mnemonics will make it easier for you to quickly remember needed information. Interviewing techniques will help you move the interview along quickly without alienating your patients. Every chapter begins with an Essential Concepts box that lists the truly take-home items of information therein. The appendices contain useful little stocking stuffers, such as "pocket cards" with vital information to be photocopied and forms that you can use during your interviews to ensure that you're not forgetting anything important.

However, if you're looking for theoretical justifications and point-by-point evidence for the efficacy of these techniques, you won't find it here. Go to one of the many textbooks of psychiatric interviewing for that. Every piece of information in this manual had to meet the following stringent standard: It had to be immediately useful knowledge for the trainee about to step into the room with a new patient.

WHAT THIS MANUAL *IS*

First, this is *only* a manual. It's not a residency or an internship. The way to learn how to interview patients is by interviewing them under good supervision. Only there can you learn the subtleties of the interview, the skills of understanding the interactions between you and your patients.

It is a tool that lends you a guiding hand in your initial efforts to interview patients. It's confusing territory. There are lots of mistakes to be made and many embarrassing and awkward moments ahead. This book won't prevent all of that, but it will catalyze the development of your interviewing skills.

It is a handbook for any beginning clinician who does psychiatric assessments as part of his or her training. This includes psychiatric residents, medical students, psychology interns, social work interns, mental health workers, nursing students, and residents in other medical fields who may need to do an on-the-spot diagnostic assessment while waiting for a consultant.

WHAT THIS MANUAL IS *NOT*

It is not a *textbook* of psychiatric interviewing. There are a number of interviewing textbooks already available (Shea 1998; Othmer 2001; Morrison 2014), my favorite being Shea's *Psychiatric Interviewing: The Art of Understanding*. Although textbooks are more thorough and encyclopedic, the drawback is that they do not guide the beginner to the essence of what he or she needs to know. Also, textbooks aren't portable, and I wanted to write something that you can carry around to your various clinical settings. That said, please buy a textbook, and have it around for those times when you want to read in more depth.

This is also not a handbook of psychiatric *disorders*. There are plenty of good ones already published, and I wrote this manual to fill the need for a brief, how-to guide to diagnosing those disorders.

Finally, it is not a *psychotherapy* manual. Doing a rapid diagnostic assessment isn't psychotherapy, although you can extend many of the skills used in the first interview to psychotherapy.

I hope that you will enjoy this book and that it will help you to develop confidence in interviewing. As you embark, remember these words of Theodore Roosevelt: "The only man who never makes a mistake is the man who never does anything." Good luck!

Introduction to the Fourth Edition

It's been 17 years since the first edition of *The Psychiatric Interview* was published. What began as a little pet project while I was a chief resident at Massachusetts General Hospital in 1995 has, surprisingly to me, become a standard text for those seeking a brief how-to manual for the psychiatric interview.

This latest edition incorporates the changes in diagnostic criteria published in DSM-5, the latest version of our field's official categorization of mental disorders. There are significant changes in how we diagnose dementia (now called major neurocognitive disorder), substance abuse, eating disorders, ADHD, and somatization disorder (which has evaporated from DSM-5). Beyond that, I did an updated literature review and made a few revisions as a result.

The Psychiatric Interview has now been translated into German, Japanese, Korean, Portuguese, and Greek. It's gratifying to me that clinicians all over the world understand the importance of active listening and of asking the right questions at the right times. Becoming a great clinician requires a lifetime of dedication. As Vince Lombardi once said, "Perfection is not attainable, but if we chase perfection we can catch excellence."

Daniel Carlat, M.D.
Newburyport, Massachusetts, 2016

Acknowledgments

For this fourth edition, as in the previous three editions, I start by thanking Dr. Shawn Shea, whose classic textbook, *Psychiatric Interviewing: The Art of Understanding*, got me interested in this topic. Dr. Shea has been a great friend and mentor throughout my career.

My father, Paul Carlat, who is also a psychiatrist, has bestowed upon me whatever personal qualities have been helpful as I work with patients. He continues to practice psychiatry, offering a unique blend of psychotherapy and medication treatment, and is a role model both for me and for many other young psychiatrists in the San Francisco Bay Area who have benefited from his supervision.

Many members of the faculty of Massachusetts General Hospital (MGH), where I did my psychiatric residency, were extremely helpful in the shaping of the manuscript. In particular, I thank the late Dr. Ed Messner, whose very practical approach to patient care was refreshing; Dr. Paul Hamburg, who taught empathy and innumerable other aspects of connecting with patients; Dr. Paul Summergrad, a consummate clinician and the director of the inpatient unit during my chief residency, who supported me in my efforts to create an interviewing course for residents; Dr. Carey Gross, who taught me much about how to rapidly make the right diagnosis for the most difficult patients; and Dr. Anthony Erdmann, who generously contributed several screening questions. In addition, special thanks go to the late Dr. Leston Havens, who was very encouraging throughout this project.

I also thank the psychiatry residents at MGH. The PGY-2 residents of the 1994 to 1995 academic year were extremely accommodating as I developed my interviewing curriculum while teaching it; the residents and psychology fellows in my own class constantly cheered me on, particularly Drs. Claudia Baldassano, Christina Demopulos, and Alan Lyman; comembers of the Harvard Gardens Club; and Dr. Robert Muller, psychologist supreme.

Finally, thanks are due to the staff of the Anna Jaques Hospital inpatient psychiatry unit, where I have "road tested" the many techniques described in this book. I especially thank Dr. Rowen Hochstedler, my former medical director at the hospital, and my friend, who is living proof that excellent mentoring can continue far beyond the reaches of academia.

Contents

Appendixes

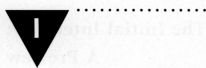

GENERAL PRINCIPLES OF EFFECTIVE INTERVIEWING

The Initial Interview: A Preview

> **Essential Concepts**
>
> **The Four Tasks**
> - Build a therapeutic alliance.
> - Obtain the psychiatric database.
> - Interview for diagnosis.
> - Negotiate a treatment plan with your patient.
>
> **The Three Phases**
> - Opening phase
> - Body of the interview
> - Closing phase

FOUR TASKS OF THE DIAGNOSTIC INTERVIEW

When you meet a patient for the first time, you know very little about her, but you know that she is suffering. (Note: Throughout this book, I switch genders when discussing theoretical patients rather than resorting to the awkward "him or her.") While this may seem obvious, this implies something that we often lose sight of. Our job, from the first "hello," is to ease our patients' suffering, rather than to make a diagnosis.

Don't get me wrong—the diagnosis is important. Otherwise, I wouldn't be subjecting you to yet another edition of this book! But diagnosis is only one step on the path of relieving suffering. And often, you can do plenty to help a patient during the first session without having much of a clue as to the official DSM diagnosis.

Since 2005, when the second edition of this book was published, psychiatry has begun to question its fixation on the value of diagnostic categories. We have come to realize that "major depression" does not imply a specific "disease" but rather a huge range of potential problems. Each of our patients present with their own versions of depression, in other words, and each version requires an individualized treatment approach. A 24-year-old woman floundering around after graduating from college a few years ago is depressed—and the solution may lie in helping her to clarify her goals. A 45-year-old public relations manager just found out his wife has been having an affair and he is depressed—the solution may be helping him to decide if he can ever trust her enough to engage in couple's therapy. A 37-year-old woman with three well-adjusted children and a good marriage says her life seems okay but she is depressed—she may need a course of antidepressants.

My point with these examples? Before you dive into the worthy project of becoming a world-class DSM diagnostician, experiment with spending much of your face-to-face patient time thinking about their lives, rather than your diagnosis of their lives. Engage your natural empathy, compassion, and intuition—because these represent the essence of psychological healing. And even as you progress through your career and have logged thousands of patient hours (as I have), always remind yourself of something that a wise colleague, Brian Greenberg, once told me: "I often put the DSM manual aside and tell myself, 'Brian, how are you going to make this person's journey easier?'"

The diagnostic interview is really about treatment, not diagnosis. It is important to keep this larger goal in mind during the interview, because if you don't, your patient may never return for a second visit, and your finely wrought *Diagnostic and Statistical Manual of Mental Disorders, Fifth Edition (DSM-5)* diagnosis will end up languishing in a chart in a file room.

Studies show that up to 50% of patients drop out before the fourth session of treatment, and many never return after the first appointment (Baekeland and Lundwall 1975). The reasons for treatment dropout are many. Some patients do not return because they formed poor alliances with their clinicians, some because they weren't really interested in treatment in the first place, and others because the initial interviews alone boosted their morale enough to get them through their stressors (Pekarik 1993). The upshot is that much more than diagnosis should occur during the initial interview: Alliance building, morale boosting, and treatment negotiating are also vital.

The four tasks of the initial interview blend with one another. You establish a therapeutic alliance as you learn about your patient. The very act of inquiry is an alliance builder; we tend to like people who are warmly curious about us. As you ask questions, you formulate possible diagnoses, and thinking through diagnoses leads naturally to the process of negotiating a treatment plan.

Build a Therapeutic Alliance

A therapeutic alliance forms the groundwork of any psychological treatment. Chapter 3, The Therapeutic Alliance, focuses on the alliance directly, and Chapters 4 to 13 provide various interviewing tips that will help you increase rapport with your patient.

Obtain the Psychiatric Database

Also known as the *psychiatric history*, the psychiatric database includes historical information relevant to the current clinical presentation. These topics are covered in Section II, The Psychiatric History, and include history of present illness, psychiatric history, medical history, family psychiatric history, and aspects of the social and developmental history. Gleaning this information is the substance of the interview, and throughout this step, you will have to work on building and maintaining the alliance. You will also make frequent forays into the next task, interviewing for diagnosis.

Interview for Diagnosis

The ability to interview for diagnosis—without sounding as if you're reading off a checklist of symptoms and without getting sidetracked by less relevant information—is one of the supreme skills of a clinician, and one that you will hone and develop over the course of your professional life. Section III, Interviewing for Diagnosis: The Psychiatric Review of Symptoms, is devoted to this skill; it contains chapters on how to memorize *DSM-5* criteria (Chapter 19) and on the art of diagnostic hypothesis testing (Chapter 20) and several disorder-specific chapters that focus on how to use screening and probing questions for each of the major *DSM-5* disorders (Chapters 22 to 31).

Negotiate a Treatment Plan and Communicate It to Your Patient

This process is rarely taught in residency or graduate school, and yet, it is probably the most important thing you can do to ensure that your patient adheres to whatever treatment you recommend. If your patient doesn't understand your formulation, doesn't agree with your advice, and doesn't feel comfortable telling you so, the interview may as well never have taken place. See Section IV, Interviewing for Treatment, for tips on the art of patient education and clinical negotiation.

THREE PHASES OF THE DIAGNOSTIC INTERVIEW

The diagnostic interview, like most tasks in life, has a beginning, a middle, and an end. Although this may seem obvious enough, novice interviewers often lose sight of it and therefore fail to actively structure the interview and control its pacing. The result is usually a panic-filled ending, in which 50 questions are wedged into the last 5 minutes.

It's true that there's a huge amount of information to obtain during the first interview, and time may feel like the enemy. Excellent interviewers, however, rarely feel rushed. They have the ability to obtain large amounts of information in a brief period, without giving patients the sense that they are being hurried along or made to fit into a preordained structure. One of the secrets of a good interviewer is the ability to actively structure the interview in its three phases.

Opening Phase (5 to 10 Minutes)

The opening phase includes meeting your patient, learning a bit about her life situation, and then shutting up and giving her a few uninterrupted minutes to tell you why she came. This is discussed in more detail in Chapter 3, because the opening phase is a crucial period for alliance building; the patient is making an initial decision as to your trustworthiness. The opening phase is based on careful, preinterview preparation, covered in Chapter 2, Logistic Preparations: What to Do Before the Interview. Attention to logistics ensures that you will be completely attuned to the relationship with your patient during the first 5 minutes.

Body of the Interview (30 to 40 Minutes)

Over the course of the opening phase, you will come up with some initial diagnostic hypotheses (Chapter 20), and you will decide on some interviewing priorities to explore during the body of the interview. For example, you may decide that depression, anxiety, and substance abuse are likely problems for a particular patient. You will map out an interviewing strategy for exploring these topics, which will include asking about the history of the present illness (Chapter 14); history of depression, suicidal ideation, and substance abuse (Chapters 22, 23, and 26); family history of these disorders (Chapter 17); and a detailed assessment of whether the patient actually meets *DSM-5* criteria (Chapters 20, 21, and 24) for each disorder. Once you've accomplished these priority tasks, you can move on to other topics, such as the social/developmental history (Chapter 18), medical history (Chapter 16), and psychiatric review of symptoms (Section III).

Closing Phase (5 to 10 Minutes)

Although you may be tempted to continue asking diagnostic questions right up to the end of the hour, it's essential to reserve at least 5 minutes for the closing phase of the interview. The closing phase should include two components: (a) a discussion of your assessment, using the patient education techniques outlined in Chapter 32, and (b) an effort to come to a negotiated agreement about treatment or follow-up plans (Chapter 33). Of course, early in your career, it will be difficult to come up with a coherent assessment on the spot, without the benefit of hours of postinterview supervision and reading. This skill will improve with practice.

> *The most tactful question in the world is still inquisitive and requests an answer. To some measure, it carries the memory of all questions that could not be answered or were shaming or damning to acknowledge.*
> Leston Havens, M.D.
> A Safe Place

Logistic Preparations: What to Do Before the Interview

Essential Concepts
- Prepare the right space and time.
- Use paper tools effectively.
- Develop your policies.

The work of psychological healing begins in a safe place, to be compared with the best of hospital experience or, from an earlier time, church sanctuary. The psychological safe place permits the individual to make spontaneous, forceful gestures and, at the same time, represents a community that both allows the gestures and is valued for its own sake.

Leston Havens, M.D.
A Safe Place

Logistic preparation for an interview is important because it sets up a mellower and less stressful experience for both you and your patient. Often, trainees are thrown into the clinic without training in how to find and secure a room, how to deal with scheduling, or how to document effectively. You'll eventually arrive at a system that works well for you; this chapter will help speed up that process.

PREPARE THE RIGHT SPACE AND TIME

Secure a Space

A space war is raging in most clinics and training programs, and you must fight to secure territory. Once secured, dig trenches, call for the cavalry, and do whatever you need to do.

I remember one early lesson in this reality: I was 2 months into my training and just finishing supervision in the Warren Building of the Massachusetts General Hospital (MGH) campus. It was 12:55 p.m., and I had a therapy patient scheduled for 1:00 p.m. in the Ambulatory Care Clinic, a building so far from Warren that it practically had its own time zone. I zigged and zagged around staff and patients in the hallways on their way to the cafeteria and rushed into the clinic by 1:05 p.m. My patient was in the waiting room and got a good view of sweat trickling down my forehead. I scanned the room schedule and found that no rooms were free. Panic set in, until the secretary pointed out that the resident who had room 825 for that hour had not yet shown up. So I led my patient to 825, and we started, 10 minutes late. Five minutes later, there was a knock on the door. I opened it, and there stood the resident and his patient. I redeposited my patient in the waiting room and scoured the list for another room.

I won't torture you with the rest of this saga. Suffice it to say, we were evicted from the next room as well, and the therapy session was, in the end, only 15 minutes long, with much humiliation on my part and good-natured amusement on my patient's.

Here are some time-honored tips on how to secure a room and what to do with it once you have it:

- **Schedule the same time every week.** Try to secure your room for the same time every week. That way, you'll be able to fit interviews into your weekly schedule routinely. When it comes to psychiatric interviewing, routine is your friend. Psychodynamic psychotherapists call this routine—the same time, the same room, the same greeting—the "frame." Making it invariable reduces distractions from the work of psychological exploration.

- **Make your room your own in some way.** This isn't easy when you only inhabit it for a few hours a week. Clinic policy may forbid this, or it may be impolite (e.g., if you're using an office that belongs to a regular staff member). If possible, put a picture on the desk or the wall, bring a plant in, place some reference books on a shelf, hang some files. The room will feel more like your space, and it will seem homier to your patient. In my current office, I have a photo of my two children on my desk. In the past, I worried that this little piece of self-disclosure could cause problems with transference. Would lonely patients envy me for having a family? Would angry patients believe that I was "bragging" by showcasing my "beautiful family"? In fact, these problems haven't occurred (at least to my knowledge)—the photo is generally a good conversation starter and, for most patients, makes me seem more human and less intimidating.

- **Arrange the seating so that you can see a clock** without shifting your gaze too much. A wall clock positioned just behind your patient works well. A desk clock or a wristwatch placed between the two of you is also acceptable. The object is to allow you to keep track of the passage of time without this being obvious to your patient. It is alienating for a patient to notice a clinician frequently looking at a clock; the perceived message is "I can't wait for the end of this interview." You do need to monitor the time, though, to ensure that you obtain a tremendous amount of information in a brief period. Actually, keeping track of time will paradoxically make you *less* distracted and *more* present for your patient, since you'll always know that you're managing your time adequately.

Protect Your Time

> *Time is but the stream I go a-fishing in.*
> Henry David Thoreau

This is not to say that you should go fly-casting with your patients (though you're usually fishing for something or other during an interview). Rather, you should protect the time you schedule for interviews, so that it has that same peaceful, almost sacred quality. How to do it?

Arrive Earlier than the Patient

You need time to prepare yourself emotionally and logistically for the interview. Compose yourself. Lay out whatever forms or handouts you'll need. Answer any urgent messages that you just picked up at your message box. Breathe, meditate, do a crossword puzzle, or whatever you do to relax.

I once observed an interviewer who was visibly anxious. He crossed and uncrossed his legs and constantly kneaded his left palm with his right thumb. Eventually, the patient interrupted the interview and asked, "Doctor? Are you all right? You look nervous." He laughed. "Oh, I'm fine," he said. And no, this was not a resident, but one of my professors.

Prevent Interruptions

There are various ways to prevent interruptions:

- Ask the clinic secretary to take messages for you.
- Ask the page operator to hold all but urgent pages.
- Put your pager on vibrate mode and only answer urgent pages.
- Sign your pages out to a colleague.

Don't Overbook Patients

Know your limits. At the beginning, it may take you an hour and a half to complete an evaluation, not including the write-up. If so, book only one patient per 2-hour slot. Obviously, your training program won't allow you to maintain such a leisurely schedule for long, but you will improve and become more efficient. Eventually, you should aim toward completing the evaluation and write-up (or dictation) in 1 hour.

Leave Plenty of Time for Notes and Paperwork

The time required for paperwork will vary, depending on both the setting and the clinician. The key is to figure out how long it takes you and then to make room for it in your schedule. Don't fall into denial. If you happen to be very slow at paperwork, admit it and plan accordingly.

I know an excellent psychiatrist who has learned from experience that he has to spend 30 minutes on charting, telephoning, and miscellaneous paperwork related to patients for every hour of clinical work he does. If he spends 6 hours seeing patients, he schedules 3 hours in the evening to take care of the collateral work. Although his hourly wage decreases, he gains the satisfaction of knowing that he's doing the kind of job he wants to do.

Now, that wouldn't work for me. I schedule slightly less time with patients so that I can finish all collateral work before I see my next appointment. The point, as Polonius said in Hamlet, is to "Know thyself, and to thine own self be true."

USE CLINICAL TOOLS EFFECTIVELY

By "clinical tools," I mean the whole array of interview forms, cheat sheets, patient handouts, and patient questionnaires. Since the last edition of this book, many of us have moved to electronic health records, so we might fill out the forms on the computer and we might e-mail patients handouts. Regardless, these tools are indispensable when you see a lot of patients every day. All of the paper versions of the tools that I discuss below are in the appendices of this manual, and you are welcome to copy and use what you want. You might find all, some, or none of them useful, or you may want to adapt them to better suit your needs.

Psychiatric Interview Long Form

This psychiatric interview long form (in Appendix B) is adapted from the one used by Anthony Erdmann, an attending psychiatrist at MGH. He takes notes on it while talking to patients and puts it in his chart.

Advantages

Use of this form ensures a thorough data evaluation and saves time, because notes can be placed directly into the chart.

Disadvantages

Some patients may be alienated if you seem more interested in completing a form than in getting to know them.

Psychiatric Interview Short Form

The short form (in Appendix B) can be used for rough notes when you are going to dictate the evaluation or write it up in a longer version later.

Advantages

This form presents less of a barrier between clinician and patient than the long form and is easy to refer to while dictating.

Disadvantages

Use of the short form may lead to a less thorough evaluation.

Psychiatric Interview Pocket Card

The pocket card (in Appendix A) is used to remind you of all the topics to cover. You can jot rough notes on a blank piece of paper or not take notes at all, if you're able to remember most information.

Advantages

The card allows maximum interaction between clinician and patient, since there is no form to fill out.

Disadvantages

Required information is not fully spelled out on the pocket card, so more use of memory is required.

Patient Questionnaire[1]

Some clinicians give their patients a questionnaire (in Appendix B) such as this one before the first meeting, to decrease the time needed to acquire basic information.

Advantages

The patient questionnaire allows more time during the first session to focus on issues of immediate concern to the patient. It may heighten the patient's sense that he is actively participating in his care.

Disadvantages

If all of the patient's answers on the questionnaire are accepted at face value, invalid information may be collected. Some patients may view filling out the questionnaire as a burden.

Patient Handouts

Patients usually appreciate receiving some written information (in Appendix C) about their disorder, and it probably increases treatment compliance.

---

[1]Adapted from the questionnaire of the late Edward Messner, M.D.

Advantages

Patient handouts increase patients' understanding of their diagnosis and give them a sense that they are collaborating in their treatment.

Disadvantages

The handouts may present more information than some patients can handle early in their treatment. Information may also be misinterpreted.

DEVELOP YOUR POLICIES

From the first appointment with a particular patient, you are entering into a relationship. You need to determine the parameters of this relationship, including issues such as how and when you can be contacted, what the patient should do in case of an emergency, who you can talk to about the patient, and how to deal with missed appointments. As you face this array of decisions, the following tips and ideas should help you devise policies that fit your personality and clinical setting.

Contacting You

You define the boundaries of the clinical relationship by setting limits on where and when patients can reach you. Do this early on; if you don't, you'll eventually suffer for it.

I found this out the hard way with my very first therapy patient during residency. She was a 40-year-old woman I'll call Sally who had panic disorder and depression. I first met her in the crisis clinic, where she came after an upsetting conversation with her father. I spoke to her for half an hour, and I gave her a follow-up appointment for the next week— and I gave her my pager number and told her that this was a way to reach me, "anytime." The next Saturday morning, over breakfast and the paper, I got my first page: "Call Sally." She was in the middle of a panic attack, which subsided after a 10-minute conversation. Later that day, as I was riding my bike, I got another page. "Call Sally." I was somewhere on a country road in Concord, Massachusetts, and far from a phone. Ten minutes later: "Call Sally. Urgent." Over the next hour, I received six pages, each sounding more urgent as the alarmed hospital operator added more and more punctuation. The last page read, "Call Sally!!! Emergency!!!!!!" When I finally found a pay phone, my heart pounding, Sally said, "Doctor! I just had another panic attack."

I felt the first hint of what I later learned was "countertransference." At the time, I called it "being pissed off." I tried to keep the irritation out of my voice as I told her she didn't have to call me every time she had a panic attack. At our next appointment, after some good supervision, I laid out some ground rules. Sally could page me only during the week between 8 a.m. and 5 p.m. Otherwise, she was instructed to go to the crisis clinic. This in itself helped decrease the frequency of her panic attacks, since it took away the reinforcement of a phone conversation with her therapist every time she panicked.

Suggestions

- Never give your home or cell phone number to patients, and consider keeping an unlisted phone number. Having made that pronouncement, I acknowledge that some of my colleagues disagree, and give patients their cell phone numbers. They do so with the understanding that they are to use that phone only under extraordinary, life-threatening circumstances. They tell me that this privilege is rarely abused and that sharing their cell phone number tells patients that you care enough about them to make sure that they can always reach you.

- You may give out your paging number, but specify the times when you're available to be paged. Don't let your life revolve around your pager. Tell your patient what to do if there is an emergency at a time when you are not available for paging. For example, he can call the crisis clinic, and you can give the clinic instructions to page you after hours if the on-call clinician judges that the situation warrants your immediate involvement.

- If you have a voice-mail system, have patients reach you there. Your voice mail is accessible 24 hours a day, and you can check it whenever you want and decide who to call back and when. Some patients will call your voice mail just to be soothed by your recorded voice.

- When you're on vacation, I suggest you sign your patients out to a clinician you know and trust, rather than have them call the crisis clinic during regular hours. That way, you can ensure that someone is prepared to deal with any impending crises. For example, you may have patients who are chronically suicidal but rarely require hospitalization and can be managed through crises with frequent outpatient support. Letting your colleague know about these patients may prevent inappropriate hospitalization. Before you go on vacation, don't forget to change your outgoing voice-mail message to tell patients how to reach your coverage. I make things easy by writing out two scripts: one for regular outgoing messages and one for vacations.

Many clinicians use e-mail as a way of contacting patients. This can be a time-saver, because you can answer quick questions without being at the mercy of the availability of your patient's cell phone or voice mail. But again, without certain ground rules, this can (and will) get out of hand. Make sure your patients know that e-mail communication is not a form of treatment. Specify what you are willing to use e-mail for. Typically, this will be limited to scheduling changes and requests for prescription refills. If you start answering more involved clinical questions over e-mail, be aware that this is part of the medical record, and you should print out a copy of any correspondence and put it in the chart. In addition, many authorities believe that HIPAA regulations require that you use an encrypted e-mail system for any electronic communication. Such systems are expensive and somewhat inconvenient, so I personally do not follow this guidance. Instead, I append a message at the end of my e-mails to patients saying: "Please be aware that e-mail communication can be intercepted in transmission or misdirected. Your use of e-mail to communicate protected health information to us indicates that you acknowledge and accept the possible risks associated with such communication. Please consider communicating any sensitive information by telephone, fax, or mail. If you do not wish to have your information sent by e-mail, please contact the sender immediately." (See *The Carlat Psychiatry Report*, October 2015 for information on a variety of encrypted methods for communicating with patients).

Contacting the Patient

Be sure to get your patient's various phone numbers (e.g., home, work, day treatment program) and e-mail (if applicable to your practice). Ask whether it's okay for you to identify yourself when you call, because some patients don't want employers or family members to know that they're in treatment. Obtain numbers of family members or close friends so that you can contact them either to gather clinical information or in emergency situations. You'll need to obtain your patient's consent for this ahead of time.

Missed Appointments

The usual practice is to tell patients that they must inform you at least 24 hours in advance of any missed appointments or they will be charged, except in emergency situations. As a salaried trainee, the financial aspects of this policy aren't relevant, but there are important clinical benefits. Patients who make the effort to show up for sessions show a level of commitment that bodes well for therapeutic success. This policy encourages that commitment.

What if a patient repeatedly cancels sessions (albeit in time to avoid paying)? First, figure out why she is canceling. Is it for a legitimate reason, or is she acting out some feelings of anxiety or hostility? Did you just return from vacation? If so, this is a common time for patients to act out a sense of having been abandoned by you.

One way to approach this issue is head-on:

> *I notice that since I returned from vacation, you've canceled three sessions in a row. What's going on? Sometimes, people get angry at their therapists.*
> *I've noticed that since we started talking about the causes of your bulimia, you've missed a lot of sessions. Should we be going a bit more slowly with these issues?*

3 The Therapeutic Alliance: What It Is, Why It's Important, and How to Establish It

> **Essential Concepts**
> - Be warm, courteous, and emotionally sensitive.
> - Actively defuse the strangeness of the clinical situation.
> - Give your patient the opening word.
> - Gain your patient's trust by projecting competence.

The therapeutic alliance is a feeling that you should create over the course of the diagnostic interview, a sense of rapport, trust, and warmth. Most research on the therapeutic alliance has been done in the context of psychotherapy, rather than the diagnostic interview. Jerome Frank, author of *Persuasion and Healing* (Frank and Frank 1991) and the father of the comparative study of psychotherapy, found that a therapeutic alliance is the most important ingredient in all effective psychotherapies. Creating rapport is truly an art and therefore difficult to teach, but here are some tips that should increase your success.

BE YOURSELF

While there is much to be learned from books and research about how to be a good interviewer, you'll never enjoy psychiatry very much unless you can find some way to inject your own personality and style into your work. If you can't do this, you'll always be working at odds with who you are, and this work will exhaust you.

CLINICAL VIGNETTE

My friend and colleague, Leo Shapiro, does both inpatient and outpatient work. He's a character, no question about it. As a patient, you either love him or hate him, but either way, what you see is what you get.

Two examples of Dr. Shapiro's unorthodox style:

1. Walking down the hallway of the inpatient unit, Dr. Shapiro spotted the patient he needed to interview next.

   "Hey, what's wrong, does your face hurt?"
   Patient: "No, my face doesn't hurt."
   Dr. Shapiro: "Well, it's killing me!"
   The patient chuckled, and the rapport was solidified.

2. The Shapiro thumb wrestling ploy

   An angry, depressed man was demanding to be discharged, prematurely according to staff reports. Dr. Shapiro agreed that discharge would be risky, partly because the patient had developed little in the way of rapport with anyone.
   Dr. Shapiro: "I understand you want to be discharged?"
   Patient: "Of course, this place is stupid, no one's helping me."
   Dr. Shapiro: "If you can beat me at thumb wrestling, I'll let you leave."
   Patient: "What?!!!"
   Dr. Shapiro (putting out his hand): "Seriously. Or are you afraid of the challenge?"
   Patient (reluctantly joining hands with Shapiro): "This is crazy."
   Dr. Shapiro: "One, two, three, go"
   Dr. Shapiro quickly wins, as he always does. "Well, I guess you have to stay another day. See you tomorrow."
   Patient (smiling, despite himself): "That's it?"
   Dr. Shapiro: "What? You wanna talk, OK, let's talk."
   A significant exchange ensued, and the patient was in fact discharged that afternoon with appropriate follow-up.
   No, I'm not endorsing the Shapiro technique. It works great for him, because that's his personality, but it would be a disaster for me, a mellow Californian at heart. The key is to be able to adapt your own personality to the task at hand—helping patients feel better.

BE WARM, COURTEOUS, AND EMOTIONALLY SENSITIVE

Are there any specific interviewing techniques that lead to good rapport? Surprisingly, the answer appears to be "no," and that is good news. A group of researchers from London have studied this question in depth and published their results in seven papers in the *British Journal of Psychiatry* (Cox et al. 1981a,b; 1988). Their bottom line was that several interviewing styles were equally effective in eliciting emotions. As long as the trainees whom they observed behaved with a basic sense of warmth, courtesy, and sensitivity, it didn't particularly matter which techniques they used; all techniques worked well.

No book can teach you warmth, courtesy, or sensitivity. These are attributes that you probably already have if you are in one of the helping professions. Just be sure to consciously activate these qualities during your initial interview.

There are, however, some specific rapport-building techniques that you should be aware of:

- **Empathic or sympathetic statements**, such as "you must have felt terrible when she left you," communicate your acceptance and understanding of painful emotions. Be careful not to overuse empathic statements, because they can sound wooden and insincere if forced.
- **Direct feeling questions** such as "How did you feel when she left you?" are also effective.
- **Reflective statements**, such as "You sound sad when you talk about her," are effective but also should not be overused, because it can seem as though you are stating the obvious.

What do you do if you don't like your patient? Certainly, some patients immediately seem unlikeable, perhaps because of their anger, passivity, or dependence. If you are bothered by such qualities, it's often helpful to see them as expressions of psychopathology and awaken your compassion for the patient on that basis. It may also be that your negative feelings are expressions of countertransference, which is discussed in Chapter 13.

ACTIVELY DEFUSE THE STRANGENESS OF THE CLINICAL SITUATION

It's easy to lose sight of the fact that an hour-long psychiatric interview is a strange and anxiety-provoking experience. Your patient is expected to reveal his or her deepest and most shameful secrets to a perfect stranger. There are several ways to quickly defuse that strangeness.

- **Greet your patient naturally.** While there are many perfectly acceptable ways to greet patients, a general rule of thumb is to act naturally, which usually means introducing yourself and shaking hands. I often engage in some small talk for the first few seconds, because many patients have a distorted view of psychiatrists as mysterious, silent types who busily scrutinize a patient's smallest gestures. Small talk undermines this projection and puts the patient at ease. Acceptable topics include the weather and difficulties arriving at the office.

Hi, I'm Dr. Carlat. Nice to meet you. I hope you were able to make your way through the maze of the hospital without too much trouble.

Ask the patient what he wants to be called, and make sure to use that name a few times during the interview.

Do you prefer that I call you Mr. Whalen, or Michael, or something else?

Using the patient's name, especially the first name, is a great way of increasing a sense of familiarity.

Caveat: Some patients (as well as some clinicians) view small talk as unprofessional. I try to size up my patient visually before deciding how to greet him or her. For example, small talk is rarely appropriate for patients who are in obvious emotional pain or for grossly psychotic patients, particularly if they are paranoid.

- **Get to know the patient as a person first.** Some patients find it awkward to reveal sensitive information to a stranger. If you sense that this is the case, you might want to begin by learning something about them as people.

Before we get into the issues that brought you here, I'd like to know a little bit about you as a person—where you live, what you do, that sort of thing.

Learning a bit about your patient's demographics at the outset has the added advantage of helping you start your diagnostic hypothesizing. There's a reason why the standard opening line of a written or oral case presentation is a description of demographics: "This is a 75-year-old white widower who is a retired police officer and lives alone in a small apartment downtown." You can already begin to make diagnostic hypotheses: "He's a widower and thus at high risk for depression. He's elderly, so at higher risk for dementia. He apparently had a career as a police officer, so probably is not schizophrenic," and so on. Knowing basic demographics at the outset doesn't excuse you from asking all the questions required for a diagnostic evaluation, but it certainly helps set priorities in the direction of inquiry.

• **Educate the patient about the nature of the interview.** Not every patient understands the nature of an evaluation interview. Some may think that this is the first session in a long-term psychotherapy. They may come into the interview with the negative, media-fed expectation of a clinician who sits quietly and inscrutably while the patient pours out his soul. Others may have no idea why they are talking to you, having been referred to a "doctor" by an internist who believes psychological factors are interfering with their medical treatment. Thus, it's helpful to begin by asking the patient if he understands the purpose of the interview and then to give him your explanation, including the expected length of time of the interview, what sorts of information you'll be asking about, and whether you will follow him for further treatment if needed.

Interviewer (I): So, Mr. Johnson, did your doctor explain the purpose of this interview?

Patient (P): She said you might be able to help me with my nerves.

I: I certainly hope I can do that. This is what we call an evaluation interview. We'll be meeting for about 50 minutes today, and I'll be asking you all sorts of questions, some about your nerves, some about your family and other things, all so I can best understand what might be causing you the troubles you've been having. Depending on your problem, we may need to meet twice to complete this evaluation, but the way our clinic works is that I won't necessarily be the one who will treat you over the long term; depending on what I think is going on, I may refer you to someone else for treatment.

- **Address your patient's projections.** Keep in mind that a lot of shame is associated with psychiatric disorders. Patients commonly project aspects of their own negative self-images onto you. They may see you as critical or judgmental. Havens (1986) recognized this and encouraged the use of "counterprojective statements" to increase the patient's sense of safety:

It may be embarrassing for you to reveal all these things to a stranger. Who knows how I'd react? In fact, I'm here to understand you and to help you.

CLINICAL VIGNETTE

Paranoid patients often project malevolent intentions onto the interviewer. In this example, the interviewer addresses these projections directly:

I: *Are you concerned about why I'm asking all these questions?*
P: *Sure. You've got to wonder—What's in it for you? How are you going to use all this information?*
I: *I'm going to use it to understand you better and to help you. It won't go any further than this room.*
P: *(Smirking) I've heard that before.*
I: *Did someone turn it against you?*
P: *You bet.*
I: *Then I can understand that you'd be careful about talking to me—you probably think I'd do the same thing.*
P: *You never know.*

With the distrust issue brought out into the open, the patient was more forthcoming throughout the rest of the interview.

GIVE YOUR PATIENT THE OPENING WORD

In one study of physicians, patients were allowed to complete their opening statements of concern in only 23% of cases (Beckman and Franckel 1984). An average of 18 seconds elapsed before these patients were interrupted. The consequence of this highly controlling interviewing style is that important clinical information may never make it out of the patient's mouth (Platt and McMath 1979).

You should allow your patients about 5 minutes of "free speech" (Morrison 2014) before you ask specific questions. This accomplishes two goals: First, it gives your patient the sense that you are interested in listening, thereby establishing rapport, and second, it increases the likelihood that you will understand the issues that are most troubling to the patient and thereby make a correct diagnosis. Shea (1998) has called this initial listening phase the "scouting period," because you can use it to scout for clues to psychopathology that you will want to follow up on later in the interview. It has also been called the "warm-up" period by Othmer and Othmer (2001), because one of its purposes is to create a comfort level between you and the patient so that the patient is not put off by the large number of diagnostic questions to come.

Of course, you have to be flexible. Some patients begin in such a vague or disorganized fashion that you will have to ask your questions right away, whereas others are so articulate that if you let them talk for 10 or 20 minutes, they will tell you almost everything you need to know.

Each clinician develops his or her own first question, but all first questions should be open-ended and should invite the patient's story. Here are several examples of first questions:

- What was it that brought you to the clinic today?
- What brings you to see me today?
- What sorts of things have been troubling you?
- How can I be of help to you?
- What can I do for you?

A somewhat different way of approaching the first question is to view it as a way of immediately exploring what that patient's goals are for the interview. Called "solution-focused interviewing," this approach is recommended by Chang and Nylund (2013).

Rather than asking "What brings you in?" or "What troubles you?" he recommends "What would make this a helpful visit?" "What would you like to see different from coming here?" This approach may work out particularly well with reluctant patients, who may not believe they have any problems in the first place.

A related question type is "the Miracle question," which goes like this: "Imagine that tonight you go to bed, like you normally do. Then, imagine that while you're asleep.... [pause)] ...a miracle happens. Imagine that because of this miracle, your depression [or whatever the patient's problem is] goes away. What will your day be like tomorrow?"

Patient: "Well, I guess I would wake up, and rather than sleep in, I'd wake up on time and get ready instead of procrastinating. Then I'd eat breakfast rather than skipping it, and at breakfast, we'd all get along better without fighting. Then I'd go to work, and I'd have more confidence, so I would say 'no' to people if they ask me to do too much...."

GAIN YOUR PATIENT'S TRUST BY PROJECTING COMPETENCE

This is always a tricky issue for novice interviewers, who often feel anything but competent. In fact, your patient usually gives you the benefit of the doubt here, because of something called "ascribed" competence. This is the competence your patient attributes to you purely because of your institutional ties. You work for Hospital X or University Y, so you must be competent. Ascribed confidence will get you through the first several minutes of the interview, but after that, you have to earn your patient's respect.

Gaining a patient's trust is easier than you might think. Even as a novice, you know much more about mental illness than your patient, and this knowledge is communicated by the kinds of questions you ask. For example, your patient tells you she is depressed. You immediately ask questions about sleep and appetite. Most patients will be impressed by your ability to elicit relevant data in this way.

Other, more prosaic ways of projecting competence include dressing professionally and adopting a general attitude of confidence. At the end of the interview, your ability to provide meaningful feedback will further cement your patient's respect.

Asking Questions I:
How to Approach
Threatening Topics

Always the beautiful answer who asks a more beautiful question.

E. E. Cummings

Over the course of the diagnostic interview, many of your questions will be threatening to your patient. The simple admission of psychiatric symptoms is humiliating for many people, as is the admission of behaviors considered by society to be either undesirable or abnormal. Such behaviors include drug and alcohol abuse, violence, and homosexuality. Beyond this, there are other behaviors that your patients may not want to admit, because they may think you will disapprove of them personally. These might include a history of noncompliance with mental health treatment, a checkered work history, or a deficient social life.

To maintain a healthy self-image, patients may lie when asked what they perceive to be threatening questions. This has been a significant problem among both clinicians and professional surveyors for years, and a repertoire of interviewing techniques has been developed to increase the validity of responses to threatening questions (Bradburn 2004; Payne 1951; Shea 1998). Good clinicians instinctively use many of these techniques, having found through trial and error that they improve the validity of the interview.

NORMALIZATION

Normalization is the most common and useful technique for eliciting sensitive or embarrassing material. The technique involves introducing your question with some type of normalizing statement. There are two principal ways to do this:

1. Start the question by implying that the behavior is a normal or understandable response to a mood or situation:

   With all the stress you've been under, I wonder if you've been drinking more lately?

   Sometimes when people are very depressed, they think of hurting themselves. Has this been true for you?

   Sometimes when people are under stress or are feeling lonely, they binge on large amounts of food to make themselves feel better. Is this true for you?

2. Begin by describing another patient (or patients) who has engaged in the behavior, showing your patient that she is not alone:

   I've seen a number of patients who've told me that their anxiety causes them to avoid doing things, like driving on the highway or going to the grocery store. Has that been true for you?

   I've talked to several patients who've said that their depression causes them to have strange experiences, like hearing voices or thinking that strangers are laughing at them. Has that been happening to you?

   It's possible to go too far with normalization. Some behaviors are impossible to consider normal or understandable, such as acts of extreme violence or sexual abuse, so don't use normalization to ask about these.

SYMPTOM EXPECTATION

Symptom expectation, also known as the "gentle assumption" (Shea 1998), is similar to normalization: You communicate that a behavior is in some way normal or expected. Phrase your questions to imply that you already assume the patient has engaged in some behavior and that you will not be offended by a positive response. This technique is most useful when you have a high index of suspicion of some self-destructive activity. A few examples follow:

- **Drug use.** Your patient has reluctantly admitted to excessive alcohol use, and you strongly suspect abuse of illicit drugs. Symptom expectation may encourage a straightforward, honest response.

What sorts of drugs do you usually use when you're drinking?

- **Suicidality.** Your patient is profoundly depressed and has expressed feelings of hopelessness. You suspect SI, but you sense that the patient may be too ashamed to admit it. Rather than gingerly asking "Have you had any thoughts that you'd be better off dead?" you might decide to use symptom expectation.

What kinds of ways to hurt yourself have you thought about?

Remember to use this technique only when you suspect that the patient has engaged in the behavior. For example, the question "What kinds of recreational drugs do you use?" may be appropriate when interviewing a young male admitted for a suicidal gesture while intoxicated, but wildly inappropriate for a 70-year-old woman being assessed for dementia.

SYMPTOM EXAGGERATION

Frequently, a patient minimizes the degree of his pathology, to fool either you or himself. Symptom exaggeration or amplification (Shea 1998), often used with symptom expectation, is helpful in clarifying the severity of symptoms. The technique involves suggesting a frequency of a problematic behavior that is higher than your expectation, so that the patient feels that his actual, lower frequency of the behavior will not be perceived by you as being "bad."

How much vodka do you drink each day? Two fifths? Three? More?
How many times do you binge and purge each day? Five times? Ten times?
How many suicide attempts have you had since your last hospitalization? Four? Five?

As is true for symptom expectation, you must reserve this technique for situations in which it seems appropriate. For example, if you have no reason to suspect that a patient has a drinking problem, asking how many cases of beer he drinks each day will sound quite insulting!

REDUCTION OF GUILT

While it is true that all the techniques in this chapter boil down to reducing a patient's sense of shame and guilt, the reduction-of-guilt technique seeks to directly reduce a patient's guilt about a specific behavior in order to discover what he has been doing. This technique is especially useful in obtaining a history of domestic violence and other antisocial behavior.

Domestic Violence

> I: *When you argue with your wife, does she ever throw things at you or hit you?*
> P: *She sure does. See this scar? She threw a vase at me 2 years ago.*
> I: *Do you fight back?*
> P: *Well, yes. I've bruised her a few times. Nothing compared to what she did to me.*

Another version of this technique is to begin by asking about other people:

> I: *Do you have any friends who push around their wives or girlfriends when they have an argument?*
> P: *Sure. They get pushed back, too.*
> I: *Have you done that yourself, pushed or hit your wife?*
> P: *Yeah. I'm not proud of it, but I've done it when she's gotten out of hand.*

Dr. Mustafa Soomro has found the following question useful: "Have you ever been in situations where fights occurred and you were affected?"

This is yet another variation on the nonjudgmental approach. If your patient answers "yes," you can flesh out whether his or her role was being a witness, a victim, or a perpetrator (Shea 2007).

Antisocial Behavior

> I: *Have you ever had any legal problems?*
> P: *Oh, here and there. A little shoplifting. Normal stuff.*
> I: *Really? What was the best thing you ever stole?*
> P: *The best thing? Well, I was into cars for a while. I spent a week cruising around in a Porsche 924, but I returned it. I was just into joyrides. Everyone was doing it back then.*

In this example, the interviewer used induction to bragging to reduce the patient's sense of guilt and lead to an admission of something more significant than shoplifting.

USE FAMILIAR LANGUAGE WHEN ASKING ABOUT BEHAVIORS

Bradburn (2004) compared two methods of asking about alcohol use and sexuality. In the first method, they used "standard" language—words and phrases such as *intoxicated* and *sexual intercourse*. In the second method, they used "familiar" or "poetic" language—the language their respondents used for the same behavior, like *getting loaded* and *making love*. They found that the use of familiar language increased reports of these behaviors by 15%.

Apparently, patients feel more comfortable admitting to socially undesirable behaviors if they feel the interviewer "speaks their language." The table below suggests various colloquial expressions to use in place of more formal language.

Using Familiar Language

Instead of	Say
Do you have a history of intravenous drug use?	Have you ever shot up?
Do you smoke marijuana?	Do you get high? Do you smoke dope?
Do you use cocaine?	Do you snort coke? Smoke crack?

Asking Questions II: Tricks for Improving Patient Recall

Essential Concepts
- Anchor questions to memorable events.
- Tag questions with specific examples.
- Describe syndromes in your patient's terms.

Uttering a word is like striking a note on the keyboard of the imagination.

Ludwig Wittgenstein

Throughout the diagnostic interview, your patient's memory will be both your ally and your enemy. Even when the desired information is not threatening in any way, be prepared for major inaccuracies and frustration if the events described occurred more than a few months ago. Nonetheless, we've all had the in-training experience of watching an excellent teacher elicit large quantities of historical information from a patient for whom we could barely determine age and sex. How do they do it? Here are some tricks of the trade.

ANCHOR QUESTIONS TO MEMORABLE EVENTS

Researchers have found that most people forget dates of events that occurred more than 10 days in the past (Azar 1997). Instead, we remember the distant past in relation to memorable events or periods (Bradburn 2004), such as major transitions (graduations and birthdays), holidays, accidents or illnesses, major purchases (a house or a car), seasonal events ("hurricane Katrina"), or public events (such as 9/11 or President Obama's election).

As an example, suppose you are interviewing a young woman with depression. You find out over the course of the interview that she has a heavy drinking history, and you want to determine which came first, the alcoholism or the depression. You could ask, "How many years ago did you begin drinking?" followed by "How many years ago did you become depressed?" but chances are you won't get an accurate answer to either question. Instead, use the anchoring technique:

> *Interviewer: Did you drink when you graduated from high school?*
>
> *Patient: I was drinking a lot back then, every weekend at least. Graduation week was one big party.*
>
> *Interviewer: Were you depressed then, too?*
>
> *Patient: I think so.*
>
> *Interviewer: How about when you first started high school? Were you drinking then?*
>
> *Patient: Oh no, I didn't really start drinking until I hooked up with my best friend toward the end of my freshman year.*
>
> *Interviewer: Were you depressed when you started school?*
>
> *Patient: Oh yeah, I could barely get up in time to make it to classes, I was so down.*

You've succeeded in establishing that her depression predated her alcoholism, which may have important implications for treatment.

TAG QUESTIONS WITH SPECIFIC EXAMPLES

In Chapter 8, you'll learn about the value of multiple-choice questions in limiting overly talkative patients. Tagging with examples is similar to posing multiple-choice questions, but it is used specifically for areas in which your patient is having trouble with recall. You simply tag a list of examples onto the end of your question.

To ascertain what medications your patient has taken in the past for depression, for example:

> *Interviewer: What were the names of the medications you took back then?*
>
> *Patient: Who knows? I really don't remember.*
>
> *Interviewer: Was it Prozac, Paxil, Zoloft, Elavil, Pamelor?*
>
> *Patient: Pamelor, I think. It gave me a really dry mouth.*

DEFINE TECHNICAL TERMS

Sometimes, what appears to be a patient's vague recall is actually a lack of understanding of terms. For example, suppose you are interviewing a 40-year-old man with depression, and you want to determine when he had his first episode:

> *Interviewer: How old were you when you first remember feeling depressed?*
> *Patient: I don't know. I've always been depressed.*

You suspect that you and the patient have different meanings of depression, and you alter your approach:

> *Interviewer: Just to clarify: I'm not talking about the kind of sadness that we all experience from time to time. I'm trying to understand when you first felt what we call a clinical depression, and by that I mean that you were so down that it seriously affected your functioning, so that, for example, it might have interfered with your sleep, your appetite, and your ability to concentrate. When do you remember first experiencing something that severe?*
> *Patient: Oh, that just started a month ago.*

6 Asking Questions III: How to Change Topics with Style

Essential Concepts
- Use smooth transitions to cue off something the patient just said.
- Use referred transitions to cue off something said earlier in the interview.
- Use introduced transitions to pull a new topic from thin air.

Interviewing a patient for the first time requires touching on many different topics within a brief period. You'll need to constantly change the subject, which can be jarring and off-putting to a patient, especially when she is involved in an important and emotional topic. Skilled interviewers are able to change topics without alienating their patients and use various transitions to turn the interview into what Harry Stack Sullivan (1970) called a "collaborative inquiry."

SMOOTH TRANSITION

In the smooth transition (Sullivan 1970), you cue off something the patient just said to introduce a new topic. For example, a depressed patient is perseverating on conflicts with her husband and stepchildren; the interviewer wants to obtain information on family psychiatric history:

Patient: John has been good to me, but I can't stand the way his daughters expect me to go out of my way to make their lives easy; after all, they're adults!

Interviewer: Speaking of family, has anyone else in your family been through the kind of depression that you've been going through?

REFERRED TRANSITION

In the referred transition (Shea 1998), you refer to something the patient said earlier in the interview to move to a new topic. For example, at the beginning of an interview, a depressed patient had briefly mentioned that he "didn't know if he could take this situation anymore." Now, well into the evaluation, the interviewer wants to fully assess suicidality:

> *Patient: My doctor tried me on some medication for a while, but it didn't do much good.*
>
> *Interviewer: Earlier, you mentioned that you didn't know how much more of this you could take. Have you had the thought that you'd be better off dead?*

INTRODUCED TRANSITION

In the introduced transition, you introduce the next topic or series of topics before actually launching into it. This transition is often begun by a statement such as "Now I'd like to switch gears ..." or "I'd like to ask some different kinds of questions now." For example, you need to quickly run through the PROS, but you don't want the patient to think that you are asking these questions because you expect that he actually experiences all of these symptoms:

> *Interviewer: Now I'd like to switch gears a little and ask you about a bunch of different psychological symptoms that people sometimes have. Many of these may not apply to you at all, and that is a useful thing to know in itself.*

Techniques for the Reluctant Patient

> **Essential Concepts**
> - Use open-ended questions and commands to increase the flow of information.
> - Use continuation techniques to keep the flow coming.
> - Shift to neutral ground when necessary.
> - Schedule a second interview when all else fails.

Occasionally, you run into the ideal patient. She's troubled and eager to talk. She briefly outlines the problems that led to her visit and then answers each of your questions in full, stopping in preparation for your next query. You find that you've gathered all the vital information in 30 minutes, and you have the luxury of exploring her social and developmental history deeply. You feel like a real therapist. Your mind is whirring, and you can't wait to dust off that copy of Freud you bought the day you got into your training program but haven't had time to look at since.

Usually, however, your patient will fall somewhere on either side of a spectrum of information flow. Either he's not saying enough or he's saying too much, and it's not his fault. The average patient has no way of knowing what information is and is not important for a psychiatric diagnosis. It's up to you to educate the patient and to steer the interview appropriately.

OPEN-ENDED QUESTIONS AND COMMANDS

You can use open-ended questions and commands to increase the flow of information. Open-ended questions can't be answered with a simple "yes" or "no."

> *What kinds of symptoms has your depression caused?*
> *What sorts of things have you done when you felt manic?*

Open-ended commands are questions altered slightly to sound more directive.

Tell me what kinds of symptoms you've had.
Describe for me some of the things you've done while you were manic.

CLINICAL VIGNETTE

The patient was a woman in her 30s who had been admitted to the hospital after an overdose. She was unhappy with the involuntary admission and initially resistant to answering questions.

> *Interviewer: I understand that you took an overdose of your medicine last week.*
> *Patient: Uh huh.*
> *Interviewer: What do you think was going on? (An open-ended question.)*
> *Patient: I don't know. (Which doesn't get anywhere.)*
> *Interviewer: Were you feeling depressed?*
> *Patient: Maybe.*
> *Interviewer: Tell me a little about how you were feeling. (An open-ended command.)*
> *Patient: There's not much to tell. I took the pills, that's all. (Still no results.)*
> *Interviewer: I really want to help you, but the only way I can do that is to understand what was going through your head when you took the pills. (Some education, combined with another, more specific, command.)*
> *Patient: I guess I thought it would be a good idea to take 'em. My husband was driving me crazy. (Now we're getting somewhere.)*

CONTINUATION TECHNIQUES

Continuation techniques can be used to keep the flow coming. These expressions encourage a patient to continue revealing sensitive information:

- Go on.
- Uh huh.
- Continue with what you were saying about…
- Really?
- Wow.

They are often combined with facilitative body language, such as head nods, persistent eye contact, holding the chin between thumb and index finger, and facial emotional response to the material. Generally, the more spontaneous and genuine your responses to reluctant patients, the more likely you are to disarm them.

NEUTRAL GROUND

Some interviews begin badly and quickly deteriorate. For example, you may have had the experience of interviewing a patient who becomes increasingly alienated as your questions become more "psychiatric." If this happens, try changing the subject to something nonpsychiatric, with the intention of sidling back into your territory once you've gained the patient's trust.

I interviewed a college student who was referred by his dean for psychological evaluation after having said he would kill himself if he was not given a better grade in a course. He was an unwilling participant and had shown up only because he was threatened with suspension if he did not.

After the first 5 minutes of the interview, it was clear that he was not interested in talking about what was going through his mind, so I shifted to relatively neutral ground.

Interviewer: So how do you like college X?
Patient: It's fine. There's a good English department.
Interviewer: Really? Any particularly interesting classes?
Patient: King Lear and the Modern World.
Interviewer: It's been a while since I read that. How is King Lear related to the modern world?
Patient: It's all about money and power. Everyone sucks up to King Lear because he has all this land to give away. It's the same way with lobbyists in Washington. Or professors at a university.
Interviewer: Is that the way it is at your college?
Patient: Of course. Professors sit in their offices, fat and happy, and students mean nothing to them. Unless they can get you to be their slave.

This led to a discussion of his frustrations with school, which in turn led to his revealing the extent of his depressive symptoms.

SECOND INTERVIEW

When all else fails, you may need to schedule a second interview. If you're not getting anywhere with the patient, no matter how many interviewing tricks you use, you may need to cut the interview short with a comment such as

> *Why don't we stop for now and meet again next week [or tomorrow, for inpatient work]. That will give you a chance to think more about the sorts of things that are bothering you, and we can take it from there.*

I've done this several times, and the patient is usually more forthcoming at the next interview. I'm not sure why this works. Maybe giving the message that I accept their reluctance paradoxically encourages them to open up, or perhaps they feel awkward about not answering questions two interviews in a row.

Of course, before you end the interview, you must feel comfortable that the patient is not at imminent risk of suicide or other dangerous behaviors.

Techniques for the Overly Talkative Patient

Essential Concepts
- Use closed-ended and multiple-choice questions to limit the flow.
- Perfect the art of the gentle interruption.
- Educate the patient about the need to move along in the interview.

> *A man does not seek to see himself in running water, but in still water. For only what is itself still can impart stillness into others.*
>
> Chuang-tzu

It was the end of a long day in the crisis clinic, and I picked up the last chart. I ushered the patient, a middle-aged woman, into the interview room. She was well groomed and socially appropriate, and she smiled warmly as she sat down. A good sign, I thought. She did not look like the sort of person who would need to be hospitalized, which is a time-consuming and exhausting process.

"How can I be of help today?" I asked.

"I am so glad I came here today," she responded. "I cannot tell you how terrible my life is. Sometimes I just don't think it's worthwhile going on. It began 21 years ago, when my first husband—a hard-drinking bastard, a real womanizer, someone I really should never have hooked up with and I wouldn't have if my parents hadn't nixed every other guy they met—and I can tell you, it was no picnic growing up in Westchester, because even though the average income is half a million, they treat their kids rotten."

A virtual torrent of information followed. For the next hour, I struggled to rein in her circumstantial and wandering stories and to get at the kernel of her complaint.

The problem with overly talkative patients is how to limit the flow of information without seeming insensitive and impatient. Cox et al. (1988), in an experimental study of interviewing techniques, found the following techniques useful for "overly expressive patients":

- Closed-ended and multiple-choice questions
- Redirecting questions to another topic
- Structuring statements regarding information required and/or clinical procedures

In general, they found that a "brisk, highly controlling style" was helpful in limiting overly expressive patients, without alienating them.

USE CLOSED-ENDED AND MULTIPLE-CHOICE QUESTIONS

Although open-ended questions should be used with most patients, they will tend to increase the talkativeness of circumstantial patients. With such patients, the open-ended approach might result in something like the following:

> *Interviewer: How have you been sleeping?*
> *Patient: Not great. Who knows, though? Do you think I've been keeping track, with each one of my kids coming at me with a different problem, one kid a day, and with work calling to ask when I'm coming back, and …*

Closed-ended questions seek brief "yes" or "no" replies or refer to a limited range of possible answers. Thus,

> *Have you been sleeping normally over the past week?*

is a closed-ended question, because it can be answered with a "yes" or "no." The following sleep question is also closed ended:

> *How many hours of sleep did you get last night?*

Although this one can't be answered with a "yes" or "no," it does refer to a limited number of possible responses, somewhere from "none" to "12 hours."

Multiple-choice questions limit answers to a greater extent than do closed-ended questions. They include a list of options for possible answers to the question, giving your patient guidance as to the level of precision expected. They are often useful in asking about the neurovegetative symptoms of depression:

> *How has your appetite been over the past few weeks:*
> *better than normal, worse than normal, or normal?*
> *What sort of sleep problem do you have? Problems*
> *falling asleep? Waking up throughout the night?*
> *Waking up too early in the morning?*

A common criticism of multiple-choice questions is that they may bias the patient toward one of your prepackaged answers. Cox et al. (1981b) examined this issue and found that patients were not biased in their replies, and that multiple-choice questions frequently yielded clear, on-topic answers.

Generally, you should sprinkle the interview with closed-ended and multiple-choice questions to rein in an overly talkative patient or with any patient with whom you have a lot of ground to cover in a very short time, such as in an emergency room evaluation. Be judicious in using these kinds of questions because some patients are alienated by them, and you risk turning a talkative patient into a terminally reluctant patient.

THE ART OF THE GENTLE INTERRUPTION

Although it may feel impolite to interrupt your patient, you're doing him no favor by letting him ramble for so long that you have insufficient time to do a proper evaluation. In some cases, you need to take charge of the interview actively. If you can accomplish this with sensitivity, you will not alienate your patient. In my experience, patients with a rambling, circumstantial style are so used to being interrupted that they barely flinch when you cut in; in fact, they often appear grateful, especially if they are working themselves into a state of anxiety or anger with their train of thought.

The gentle interruption is also known as a "redirecting statement" (Cox et al. 1988), and it comes in various guises.

In the **empathic interruption**, you add an empathic statement to soften the blow:

> *I can tell that this situation's been really hard for you to*
> *deal with. Have you been drinking lately, to cope with it?*

In the delaying interruption, you assure the patient that her topic is important and that you'd like to come back to it later:

> *I can see you feel strongly about your daughter's*
> *school troubles, and that's something we can talk*

> *about later, but right now I need to ask you about some*
> *of those signs of depression you were experiencing.*
> *Was your appetite normal through all this?*

Of course, there's also a note of empathy in that delaying statement.

The **educating interruption** incorporates a structuring statement in which you educate the patient about the sorts of questions you have yet to ask and the time constraints you're both working under. Usually, this is done only after you've used the other two interruptions several times with no results.

> *I'm sorry, but I need to interrupt you again. We have*
> *about 20 minutes left and a lot of ground to cover,*
> *including your treatment history, your family back-*
> *ground, and your medical history, and I want to make*
> *sure we have time at the end to talk about some medi-*
> *cation changes. You can help by trying to answer the*
> *questions directly and not getting too sidetracked. How*
> *does that sound?*

or,

> *It's important that I learn more about how you've been*
> *eating and sleeping so that I can tell whether you're*
> *suffering from a clinical depression, so I may continue*
> *to interrupt you to get that important information.*

or, more simply,

> *We really have a lot of ground to cover over the next*
> *half hour, so I'm going to have to ask you a lot of ques-*
> *tions. This may mean some interruptions, okay?*

Techniques for the Malingering Patient

Essential Concepts
Rule out malingering in
- Patients on disability
- Patients involved in litigation related to a psychiatric condition
- Patients seeking a prescription for a controlled substance during the initial interview

As you begin to put more and more years of practice under your belt, you will increasingly begin to recognize that some of your patients are faking their symptoms for secondary gain. Nobody knows how common this is, and it probably is pretty uncommon, but you will need to know how to recognize such patients and to "smoke them out." This chapter provides you some helpful techniques.

But before proceeding, make sure not to confuse malingering with "factitious disorder," or Munchausen's syndrome. Munchausen's involves the self-infliction of actual pain or injury with no clear secondary gain being served. Such patients may be motivated by unconscious psychodynamic motivations, and while they, like malingerers, lie about their symptoms, the ultimate treatment approach is different, because Munchausen's represents a recognized psychiatric syndrome unto itself, while malingering is just lying, plain, and simple.

CLINICAL VIGNETTE

A 34-year-old single man presented to me after having been referred by employee health at his manufacturing company. He appeared somewhat disheveled and launched into a narrative about a work situation, saying that "It all started on June 6, when this foreman called me into his office." As he began describing the episode, I reached over for my pen and clipboard. He responded to my movement with a dramatic startle response, and then explained, "I don't know what that is, it's been happening ever since that day in June." On my prompting, he described in great detail a series of events leading to his current short-term medical disability, including precise dates and names of all parties involved. During the review of psychiatric symptoms, when asked about his memory and concentration, he said, "I can't remember a single thing since June; I can't even read."

Obviously, there are a number of clues to malingering here. The "startle response" was exaggerated to the point of looking like a convulsion, and his self-described concentration problems were undermined by his masterful ability to describe the "traumatic" event at work. Over time, he failed to respond to any of the medications usually helpful for PTSD, and once he was approved for long-term disability, he stopped coming to appointments. The *coup de grace* was failure to pay his bill because of bankruptcy!

The first step in correctly diagnosing malingering is to have a high index of suspicion that it exists. All of the following patient categories are red flags for possible malingering:

- Any patient on any form of disability, whether through work or public insurance
- Any patient involved in litigation having to do with the psychiatric illness
- Any patients who, early on in the appointment, indicate that they are hoping to leave the appointment with a prescription for a controlled medication

I don't mean to sound heartless; in my experience, the majority of patients on disability are genuinely disabled, and litigation is often legitimate. But if you raise your malingering antennae with these types of patients, you'll rarely find yourself duped.

INTERVIEWING CLUES TO MALINGERING (AND STRATEGIES FOR RESPONDING)

The Tale Is Just Too Perfect

All of the symptoms are revealed in near perfect DSM-5 order. The quality of the symptoms is textbook in the sense that they are presented in the way you might if you had read their descriptions but hadn't actually experienced them.

Suggested strategies: Be extra careful not to "lead" these patients through symptoms as you might to with other new patients in the interest of time. Keep questions open ended. If you suspect that they are trying to sell you on a diagnosis, throw them a little off-balance by asking something that they are unlikely to have read much about, for example, "Did either of your parents have these PTSD symptoms?" Depending on what the answer is, act mildly surprised, saying, "That's odd, in my experience it's very unusual for the parents of someone with PTSD to have had it as well; are you sure?" The malingerer will tend to alter her answers as she feels it suits your expectations: "Well, that's only what my brother said; I always thought they were pretty normal, and I don't think they ever saw a psychiatrist."

The Tale Is too Vague

If you come across as pretty savvy in your questioning (which you hopefully will after reading this chapter!), many malingering patients will worry that they will imminently "slip up" and reveal their ruse. Such patients may resort to answering questions so vaguely that they *can't* be wrong, for example, "It's hard to say how I've been sleeping; it's been really loud outside my window lately, and sometimes when I wake up, I can't tell how long I slept."

Suggested strategies: Use extremely closed-ended questions to nail them down (e.g., see Chapter 8). If that doesn't work, precede questions with obvious leads, like, "In my experience, patients with panic attacks have tingling in their lips, has that been true?" If previously vague answers become precise with such leading, you have a pretty big clue to malingering.

The Symptoms Are Unrealistic

Dr. Philip Resnick, a forensic psychiatrist with special expertise in evaluating malingering patients, emphasizes the importance of understanding the usual characteristics of psychiatric symptoms and then comparing them to the patient's description. For example, in insanity defense cases, defendants will often say that voices have told them to do illegal things.

For example, Dr. Resnick points out that studies of genuine auditory hallucinations have shown that "66% to 88% of patients report that their voices come from outside their head; only 7% of auditory hallucinations are vague or inaudible." Furthermore, she points out that "auditory hallucinations are intermittent rather than continuous. One third of patients who have hallucinations report having command hallucinations; the majority of persons who have command hallucinations do not always obey them." And while up to a third of AH come in the form of questions, they are usually chastising rather than information seeking (Shea 2007).

Using this information, you should ask careful, detailed questions about the nature of patients' hallucinations when you suspect malingering.

> *Interviewer: Why is it so hard for you to stop shoplifting?*
> *Patient: These voices tell me to do it.*
> *Interviewer: Do the voices tell you exactly what to do?*
> *Patient: Yes, they say, "Go into Staples and take the software program."*
> *Interviewer: Are the voices inside your head?*
> *Patient: Yeah—they're like a part of me.*
> *Interviewer: Do they ask you questions?*
> *Patient: Yeah, like "How much is it worth?" Or "What time is the store open?"*

In this case, the interviewer strongly suspected the patient was malingering, particularly since there had been no prior history of psychosis in the patient's history, before his arrest for shoplifting.

"Nothing Works, Doc."

If you have established that a series of standard treatments have been tried and that they have all failed, this may simply mean that the patient has a treatment-resistant condition (which certainly happens legitimately), but it may represent an ongoing effort to keep the disability payments coming.

Suggested strategies: Asking in-depth questions about medication and psychotherapy trials will give you a better sense of whether your patient was actually compliant with anything (e.g., as a rule of thumb, you should establish at least a 4-to 6-week duration of antidepressant treatment or at least eight sessions of therapy). If they have tried the usual treatments and haven't gotten better, make sure to offer more aggressive treatment. Such offers can be very informative, as with one of my patients who declined trials of several alternative antidepressants, citing vague reasons. I explained that it would be difficult for me to continue filling out his disability forms if he didn't accept needed treatment; this turned out to be his last visit with me.

"I Heard About This Thing Called 'Klonopin' From A Friend Who Has What I Have."

Prescription substance abusers (or pushers) have to get their supply somehow, and a favorite method is to go doctor hopping until they find someone who writes the desired prescription. Red flags here include the following:

- The patient asks for the controlled medication very early in the evaluation.
- The patient quickly insists that he has tried every other potential nonaddictive treatment option and that they either have not worked or have caused intolerable side effects.
- The patient says he has tried a friend's or relative's medication.
- The patient has a history of alcohol or drug abuse.

Suggested strategies: Say, "Are you aware that (Drug X) is a very dangerous and addictive medication?" A drug seeker may respond in several different ways. He may make a big show of being surprised and say, "Really?" He may appear unfazed and smoothly respond, "I know people say it's addictive, but I've never had a problem with it." No particular response is diagnostic of malingering, but it may help sway you in one direction or another. Another helpful technique is to ask to speak to prior prescribers, be they primary care doctors, nurse practitioners, or psychiatrists. Any hedging or hesitation in response to this entirely reasonable request is cause for suspicion.

Techniques for the Adolescent Patient[1]

> **Essential Concepts**
> * Involve the family.
> * Overcome the "I don't know" syndrome.
> * Develop strategies for asking about drugs, sex, and conduct problems.

> *Don't laugh at a youth for his affectations; he is only trying on one face after another to find his own.*
> Logan Pearsall Smith

There are three reasons to include a chapter on adolescents in a book otherwise devoted to adult psychopathology: (a) Child and adolescent treatment is a part of most general training programs; (b) many primarily "adult" clinicians are called on to evaluate adolescents; and (c) many "adult" patients are still struggling through late adolescence, which begins during the later teen years and extends to the early 20s. If you can master the techniques of evaluating adolescents, you will find yourself using these same techniques for many of your adult patients, of *any* age.

THE FAMILY INTERVIEW

Your initial interview with an adolescent will usually include family members for at least part of, and sometimes all of, the session. Adolescents are great minimizers and deniers, and you often will need to interview the family separately to ascertain the presence of any problem at all. In addition, many psychiatric disorders in adolescents are strongly related to family issues, with family dynamics sometimes contributing significantly to them (e.g., oppositional defiant disorder, depression) and at other times being the cause of

---

[1]With contributions from David Sorenson, M.D., and Alan Lyman, M.D.

family strife (e.g., attention deficit hyperactivity disorder [ADHD]). Finally, treatment can rarely happen without the consent and cooperation of family members.

Thus, for the first appointment, plan to invite the entire family into your office. Usually, I walk out to the waiting room and greet the patient with an introduction and hand-shake and then face the family, saying, "Why don't we all go in for the first part of the hour, then maybe I can have some time to chat with _____ afterward."

Once in the office, allow the family to decide where to sit, and then shut up and listen for a while, just as you would with your adult patients. If there is some initial silence, you can get things going with questions such as

> *What brings us all together today?*
> *What sort of issues have been coming up?*

or, more simply,

> *Okay, who wants to do the talking?*

A parent usually begins, and it is important that you listen closely, because a family's desires may be quite different from what you suspected or from what you can provide.

CLINICAL VIGNETTE

Two parents brought in their 17-year-old son for an evaluation. Once in the office, the mother's first words were, "I want you to commit my son for his drug addiction."

The son, taken aback, turned to her and said, "Are you crazy?"

What developed was that the parents had suspected the son of drug use but had told him that this was a family therapy meeting to "work out some family issues." The mother's expectation was that the clinician would immediately have a police officer escort the patient from the office to a substance abuse treatment facility. The clinician explained that this was not possible and went on to explain the state's legal criteria for involuntary commitment. Eventually, the adolescent agreed to outpatient treatment of substance abuse and depression.

Allow at least 5 minutes of free speech, in which you simply listen to family members discussing the perceived problem. Aside from clueing you into diagnostic possibilities, this will allow you to understand the communication style and family dynamics. After listening for a few minutes, you will want to jump in with various questions to ascertain elements of the psychiatric and social history. It is important to adopt a neutral attitude so as not to appear that you are taking the parents' side. If the parents constantly speak over the patient (or vice versa), make a corrective comment, such as

> Everyone obviously has a lot of feelings about this issue, but it is important that I get a chance to hear everyone's viewpoint without too much interrupting.

After a period of time, you will want to talk to the adolescent alone.

> I enjoyed meeting you, and now, I'd like to talk about some things with Matthew. Afterward, we'll get back together and discuss what we've talked about.

THE INDIVIDUAL INTERVIEW

Initial Questions and Strategies

How much time should you devote to the individual interview? There are no hard-and-fast rules. A full hour of individual discussion may be appropriate for a sensitive and sophisticated 14-year-old adolescent with depression, whereas an angry and involuntary 17-year-old adolescent with conduct disorder may be able to tolerate no more than 5 minutes alone with you. The more verbal and engaged the patient seems, the more time you will want to allot for your individual interview with her.

So there you are, in the room alone with your adolescent patient. Clinicians who spend most of their time with adults often freeze at this point. What do you say to a 15-year-old, who may feel quite awkward and embarrassed, especially now that his parents have left the room?

You want to avoid awkward gaps in the conversation as much as possible, which may involve doing more talking than you normally do. Some degree of self-disclosure may be acceptable too, to build rapport. You can start with some tension-relieving statements such as:

> *Okay. Now I get to hear your side of the story.*
> *We have a half hour or so to talk confidentially now.*
> *I hope you'll feel comfortable telling me your side of what's been going on at home.*

If the family discussion was heated, react to that in some way:

> *Whew, things got pretty hot there; what do you think?*

Remember that adolescents may have had no prior experience with a professional who asks very personal questions. Thus, it may be helpful to begin with a comment such as

> *Do you mind if I ask you some personal questions?*
> *I may ask some questions that you're uncomfortable answering, and you don't have to answer if you don't want to.*

At some point during the interview, say something about the limits of confidentiality. Relay the statement with terms such as "worry":

> *I won't tell your parents about anything you say unless I'm really worried that your life might be in danger.*

Later, before you bring the family back in, ask

> *Is there anything you don't want me to tell your parents?*
> *Is it okay if I tell your parents about these things?*

If they say "yes," follow up with

> *Do you want to tell them or do you want me to?*

This way, you're maximizing your patient's sense of control.

"I Don't Know" Syndrome

Adolescents tend to have difficulty describing their internal emotional state. Sometimes, this is because they don't want to seem vulnerable; other times it's because their emotional vocabulary is underdeveloped. Thus, asking direct questions about feelings is likely to lead to the following type of exchange:

> *Interviewer: Have you been feeling depressed?*
> *Patient: I don't know.*
> *Interviewer: Have you been feeling angry?*
> *Patient: I don't know.*
> *Interviewer: How have you been feeling?*
> *Patient: Okay, I guess.*

How does one get beyond the "I don't know" syndrome? One way is to give the patient permission to plead the fifth:

> *Look, if you really don't know something, that's fine. But if you don't want to tell me something, that's okay too. Just say, "I don't want to say."*

Another strategy is to ask the "fly on the wall" question:

> *If I were a fly on the wall when you get into one of your moods, what would I see?*

or, a slight variation,

> *What would your friend look like if he looked like you in one of your moods?*

These questions invite the patient to describe his behavior, a less threatening proposition than describing a subjective state.

A third strategy is to rely on the defense mechanism of displacement. Ask your patient if he has any friends with problems:

> *Do you have any friends who are in trouble? What's going on with them?*

This might lead into an elaborate discussion of a friend's antisocial or suicidal behavior, which may actually be autobiographical.

Topics to Cover

Often, the trick with adolescents is to get them talking, much less getting them to reveal personal information. The best strategy is to adopt an attitude of curiosity and respect; a sense of humor is always a plus.

Most adolescents are interested in music, so this is as good a place to start as any.

> *Do you like music? Who do you like?*

Chances are that you will have never heard of their favorite group. You could respond with

> *I have no idea what kind of music that is. Me, I like jazz and, I'm ashamed to admit, Barry Manilow.*

If you're square and goofy, and most of us over 30 are, admit it. This is disarming to most adolescents and is better than trying to pose as "cool."

Asking about School and Other Activities

Other questions that help open up a shut-down adolescent include questions about school, friends, and interests. Each line of inquiry can also serve as a jumping-off point for diagnostic questions.

> *Where do you go to school?*
> *What's that school like?*
> *Is it fun?*
> *Is it easy?*
> *What are the other kids like there?*
> *Who do you hang out with?*

After asking these nonthreatening questions, ask about grades. If his grades are low or if he looks disappointed in his grades, follow up with

> *Is that the same as you've always done, or have your grades changed recently?*

A change in grades may signal the onset of depression or involvement with substance abuse. You might also ask

> *Are there any particular subjects that are hard?*

The *DSM-5* classifies learning disorders under the traditional categories of reading, writing, and arithmetic, and you can pick up a hint of a learning disorder by asking this question. However, children are usually diagnosed with a learning disability long before their teenage years.

What do you do with your time after school?
Are you involved in any extracurricular activities, like
sports or clubs?
What do you enjoy doing the most?

Besides being good questions for opening up your patient and establishing rapport, these are good screening questions for depression. Withdrawal from social activities is a common feature of teenage depression. Conversely, the patient who expresses clear interest and excitement in *any* activity is less likely to be depressed.

How many hours of TV do you watch on the average
school night?
How many hours do you spend on the computer?

This gives another indication of how socially involved your patient is.

Asking about Drugs and Alcohol

Using the techniques discussed in Chapter 4 is helpful in communicating a nonjudgmental attitude when asking about drug use. Thus, you can use normalization:

I hear there's a lot of drinking and drug use at your
school. Do you know anyone who uses drugs?
You read in the paper that 90% of kids use drugs these
days. Do you ever use drugs?

or symptom expectation:

How often do you have a drink?
What drugs do you use?

Other patients respond quite well to a direct query:

Do you drink or use drugs?

Asking about Sex

Although asking about sex is important when interviewing adolescents, use judgment and common sense in determining when such questions are appropriate. If your rapport is shaky, you may want to delay such questions for follow-up visits, or you may decide not to raise the questions at all. It's vitally important that any questions about sex *not* be seen by your patient as idle or lurid interest, but rather that they are seen as an essential component of your psychiatric evaluation. A sexual history is important for a variety of psychiatric and medical issues, including assessing risk for AIDS, discovering a history of sexual abuse, and assessing the presence of sexual acting-out as a symptom of depression, mania, substance abuse, or other disorder.

A good way to approach this uncomfortable topic is to begin talking about "romance" rather than "sex."

> *Do you have any romantic relationships?*
> *How long have you been seeing this person?*
> *What's his/her name?*
> *What do you like about_____?*

Now that you've given a human face to the relationship, you can introduce the topic of sex:

> *Would you feel comfortable if we talked about your sex life?*
> *Are you sexually active?*
> *Are you using protection?*
> *Do you know about AIDS?*
> *Do you ever do things sexually that you later regret, like not using protection or having sex with people you don't know very well?*

You can also approach sexuality by embedding it in a list of health-related questions:

> *I want to ask a few questions about your health:*
> *Do you get headaches?*
> *Stomachaches?*
> *Do you have sexual problems?*
> *Are you sexually active?*
> *Do you smoke?*
> *Do you use drugs or alcohol?*

If it seems appropriate, ask about sexual orientation:

> *Have you ever wondered whether your sexual feelings are normal?*
> *Do you ever think that your feelings about sex are different from other kids' feelings?*

Note that neither of these questions uses terms such as *sexual orientation* and *sexual identity*, either of which may confuse or alienate adolescents.

Asking about Conduct Problems

Conduct disorder and oppositional defiant disorder are common reasons for referral, and you'll often be faced with the task of getting patients to admit to illegal behavior. Usually, the parents will have disclosed such behavior during the family meeting. A good way to begin a private interview in such circumstances is as follows:

> It looks like your mom feels there's been a lot of stealing (or whatever alleged behavior), and I have no way of knowing if it's true, but if you were stealing, I'm sure there was a good reason for it. Maybe it was the only way you could get something? Or maybe your friends challenged you to do it?

or, more simply,

> Do you know what your parents are saying about what you've been doing?

If the rapport is good, and you don't mind using some humor, use the "inducing to brag" approach:

> So, I hear you're an excellent thief. What's the best thing you've stolen?

Remember that you aren't asking these questions just to get your patient to confess to bad behaviors; rather, you're primarily interested in finding out why he does these things. Is it peer pressure? A way of expressing anger toward his parents? A symptom of a manic episode? Follow up on an admission of antisocial behaviors with questions designed to address these topics.

Interviewing Family Members and Other Informants

11

Essential Concepts
- Try to have some contact with informants as part of all your initial evaluations.
- Develop an efficient approach to asking informants questions about your patient.
- Be prepared to provide basic psychoeducation to informants.

Interviewing a patient's informants—that is, their family members, friends, coworkers, etc.—is such a crucial part of many psychiatric evaluations that some clinicians will not see patients unless they agree to an informant meeting at some point during the treatment. In my experience, it is not always necessary, but when I have bothered to make it happen, it has always added something of value to my understanding of patients.

Before getting into specific suggestions, I have found it useful to think about the following three goals for interacting with family members and other informants:

1. Let the family know they are not alone.
2. Provide support and allow informants to vent.
3. Instill hope for change (adapted from Mueser and Glynn 1999).

HOW TO BROACH THE ISSUE OF TALKING TO INFORMANTS

I usually ask something like:

"As part of my evaluation of patients, I find it helpful to talk to someone else involved in your life. Would that be okay with you?"

Most patients will agree to this and will typically be impressed that you care enough to go that extra mile in conducting your evaluation. Assuming they agree, you should figure out who would be the best person to talk to—a parent, a significant other, a roommate, a friend, etc.

Sometimes patients will decline having an informant become part of the treatment, which is certainly their right. But it's helpful to find out the root of their discomfort. At times, it may be that there is something they want to hide from you, such as drug use or other behaviors at odds with their recovery. But other times, the reasons are understandable.

CLINICAL VIGNETTE

I had seen a man in his 30s for a couple of years for depression, which had gradually improved with treatment, but he continued to complain of not feeling very fulfilled with his life, and he qualified for the diagnosis of dysthymia. He acknowledged that one of the major issues in his life was the fact that his wife wanted to have more children but he didn't. Several times, I had encouraged him to bring his wife into a meeting—not for couples therapy, but in order to better understand the nature of their relationship so that I could help him in therapy. He eventually said that she would be able to attend our next session. But he came alone.

"Where's your wife?" I asked, surprised.

"I thought a lot about it, and I agreed that it might be helpful for her to come in to the session. But then I realized that this is *my* time with you."

Ultimately, *my* ready acceptance of his decision strengthened our alliance and improved the quality of our therapy.

BE READY WITH A LIST OF QUESTIONS

Your patient has shown up with his mother as you requested. What kinds of questions are you going to ask? You may feel that the pressure is on, since this may be the only time you will have to interview the informant. Therefore, it's best to be ready with a list of questions.

As with interviewing patients, when interviewing families, you'll want to start with an open-ended approach and then drill down to specific questions.

I'll often start by asking, "How do you think Nancy has been doing?" Some informants will arrive brimming with a wealth of specific and useful information, but others might answer more sparsely, with something like, "She's been okay. Sometimes she gets nerved up, but then she takes her happy pills and seems better."

In this case, the informant is not speaking your clinical language and needs education about the specific kind of information you are looking for.

Murray-Swank et al. recommend the following series of questions for informant interviews:

1. "What do you think has caused [name] to have these problems?"
2. "Has anybody ever given you a diagnosis for his/her problems?" (If they have been told of a diagnosis, it is useful to follow up with a question such as "What is your understanding of what that diagnosis means?")
3. "Are there things that make things better for [name]?"
4. "Are there things that make things worse?"

These kinds of questions allow you to teach the informant the kind of vocabulary that you will find most useful in tracking your patient's progress.

Going back to our case of nerved-up Nancy, you might say, "I think when you said that Nancy gets 'nerved up,' she is having what we think of as a panic attack, and that the 'happy pill' is Ativan, an anxiety medicine that helps her get over her panic problem." This type of psychoeducation may ultimately help your patient understand when to use her medication appropriately because it puts her and her informant on the same page.

Specific pieces of information that you might want to obtain (depending on the specific problem) include the following:

- Suicidality
- Violence
- Ability to function day to day
- Do they go to work?
- Do they *do* anything, or just sit on the couch all day long?

- Do they sleep?
- What do they eat?
- Are they concentrating OK?
- Have they always been this way, or is this a recent change?

Another way to help you organize your questioning is to try to ascertain the typical day in the life of your patient.

"Mrs. Smith, when I see your husband, it is only for about a half hour every month or so—I see only a tiny slice of his life. I'd like to know more. Beginning with when he wakes up in the morning, what is a typical day like in your husband's life?"

WHAT TO DO WHEN AN INFORMANT IS CONFRONTATIONAL

Sometimes, when a family member pops in, they are doing so because they are not particularly happy with how the patient is doing and they may be wondering if you are competent. If I sense this is true, I will meet the issue head-on.

"How do you think I've been doing with Nancy? Do you think I've been helping her at all? Am I the best doctor for her? Do you have any ideas for how I might be able to help her more?"

Obviously, you are not necessarily asking for a medication consultation from a layperson, but you'd be surprised what comes out. In one situation, I had treated a woman with a series of antidepressants. She was currently on Celexa, and I thought she was doing reasonably well on it. When her husband came to a session, it was clear that he was dissatisfied with her treatment.

"I don't think she's doing very well on this medicine," he said. "My sister is taking Paxil and she's doing great."

I had no problem with Paxil—to me, it was just one of a dozen or so equally effective antidepressants, but psychologically, it appeared to be what both the husband and my patient wanted, so I prescribed it, and the patient did well—no doubt with a large placebo component at play.

WHEN AN INFORMANT IS "ANTIMEDICATION"

Occasionally, a patient will tell me that a family member disapproves of medication treatment. If I believe that the medication is effective and necessary, I will strongly encourage an informant meeting. Sometimes, I will simply pick up the phone then and there, with the patient's permission.

At times, the informant is responding to sensationalized media reports of the dangers of psychiatric drugs, and a short meeting will help set his or her mind at ease. Other times, the informant is adamant that medications are the wrong approach, and if I feel that the patient is stable and might do well with a trial off meds, I'll readily agree to a gradual taper. In my experience, in the majority of such cases, both the patient and the informant return to my office within several months to request a medication resumption—but that is not always the case.

Sometimes, it may seem that an informant is "antimed," when in fact he or she is anti-ineffective med.

For example, one patient with bipolar disorder had literally been on every psychiatric medication that I knew of over the course of his life—I was the latest in a long line of psychiatrists. The mother, supposedly antimedication, came in and said, "I'm tired of Jack being a guinea pig. You doctors keep putting him on all these medications, and I think they make him really tired."

I asked her if any medication had worked for him. "The only medication that really works for him is lithium." Paradoxically, I had discontinued lithium several months earlier. So the informant who was billed as "antimed" ended up convincing me to put the patient back on a medication with a pretty hefty side effect burden, but it ended up being relatively effective.

WHAT DO INFORMANTS WANT INFORMATION ABOUT?

In my experience, informants frequently come into a meeting with one or more of the following underlying thoughts and worries.

- Are you going to screw around with the medications that have kept my loved one stable?
- Are you going to blame me for the patient's problems?
- Are you going to give me a bunch of new responsibilities?
- Are you a competent doctor?

- Are you going to be evaluating *my* mental health?
- Is this couples or family therapy?

There's no specific answer to each of these concerns, but it's helpful to review this list before you meet with an informant. During your conversation, you may well pick up on one of these possible concerns and then you can address it.

HOW TO DEAL WITH PRIVACY ISSUES IN THE AGE OF HIPAA

The Health Insurance Portability and Accountability Act (HIPAA) actually gives you *more*, not less, latitude in sharing patient information with other health care providers. Once your patient signs a HIPAA form, you are allowed to talk to therapists or other doctors without getting specific permission each time. However, HIPAA does not allow you to talk to family members without consent. The exception is when the patient's life is in danger.

What happens when a family member calls *you*? Can you talk to them? Yes, you can, as long as you are a recipient of information only. But they often have the misconception that they can't talk to you at all without a signed release. When an informant calls, I say, "I can listen to anything you have to say, but I won't be able to share anything your wife has told me without her consent."

I try to get the informant's agreement that I can tell the patient about the phone call and about the information I received. Sometimes, the informant is scared of the patient's possible reactions. A typical scenario is a wife calling about a husband who I am treating individually. The wife tells me that her husband had been drinking more and becoming verbally abusive. She may be terrified that if I share this phone call with the husband, he will become more abusive toward her. Obviously, if you believe that the informant is in imminent danger from your patient, you are duty bound to intervene, regardless of consent forms. But in most cases, these are judgment calls. If I feel that the information is so crucial that it will affect treatment (such as the revelation that a patient is a drug abuser), I may sometimes insist that the informant agrees to be named, because in my experience the patient figures out where I got the information pretty quickly.

INPATIENT WORK

Dealing with informants when you are doing inpatient work carries its own challenges and therefore merits a separate section of this chapter. Here is a typical inpatient informant scenario:

It's 10 a.m., and you have been scurrying around the unit trying to get your work done quickly, because you have to be at the outpatient clinic by 1 p.m. You look at your index card, and there are eight patients on your list. You have to talk with each one, meet with nurses and social workers, and write a note.

Robert Jones is next. A 23-year-old, he was admitted to the hospital 3 days ago after an apparent suicide attempt by overdose. But after having evaluated him, you feel certain that he is not truly suicidal. You found out that his "overdose" was on fifteen 1-mg pills of Klonopin—hardly enough to do much damage, especially considering that his normal prescription was 3 mg per day. The "overdose" came immediately after a telephone call with his ex-girlfriend during which she refused to consider renewing their relationship. Distraught, he took the pills and then immediately called both his father and 911. Within 10 minutes, he was in the local emergency room, from where he was admitted to the psychiatric unit. Over the course of the past 3 days, you and the rest of your team have determined that he was not suicidal and developed an outpatient treatment plan involving a referral to a local clinic that better integrates psychotherapy and psychopharmacological treatment.

Today, you walk into his room to say your goodbyes and to make sure that he understands his discharge plan. But you are surprised to see three people in the room, who turn out to be his two parents and his sister. The first question from the father is, "Are you really discharging him? After only 3 days? He just tried to kill himself!"

What do you do? A long meeting will throw your schedule off—but clearly, the family deserves to have some significant contact with their loved one's psychiatrist. Although from your perspective, this patient is one of a long list of people you must help, for the family there is only one person on their list—their loved one. Empathizing with the family will go a long way toward helping you do the right thing.

The *wrong* way to respond would be: "I'm sorry, but I don't have time for a meeting right now—but I can set up a time for you to speak with the social worker or one of the nurses." To the family, the underlying message is, "I don't really care," or "I don't have time for you," or "Your loved one's issues are not important enough to require my time."

Instead, no matter how hurried you feel, take a deep breath, smile, and say, "I'm really glad we are having a chance to meet." Make sure to find a place to sit down, because nothing says "rushed" more than a meeting while standing. Next, explain your time constraints apologetically. "I wish we had a good hour to talk about Robert, but today unfortunately, I can only meet for about 10 minutes. I'm really sorry about this, but I also think we can get a lot done to help you understand what's going on with Robert in those 10 minutes. And if you have any other questions, I'll arrange for you to meet with our social worker."

Psychoeducation

What are you realistically going to be able to accomplish in those measly 10 minutes? Primarily, you are going to be educating the family about the purposes and the limitations of inpatient psychiatric treatment. Families often think that psychiatric hospitalizations are meant to provide a definitive "answer" to a problem that has been going on for years. They may expect that you will come up with the perfect medication and that you will fix a wide range of problems, such as family dynamics issues, work problems, social problems, or school problems. If so, they need you to educate them about the realities of inpatient admissions:

"In the past, hospitalizations went on for a long time, sometimes many months. But these days, they are brief, and our goal is to solve the immediate crisis and to make sure patients are safe before they leave. We also work hard on setting up a good outpatient program, because that is where the work of healing takes place—over the long term, out in the real world."

Some clinicians will also mention that ever-present big white elephant in the room—the insurance company: "Unfortunately, insurance companies will no longer pay for admissions longer than a few days, unless the patient will be clearly unsafe if discharged."

This is a card you don't want to play too much, however, because the family may get the message that you are discharging the patient prematurely because you are not getting paid.

Learning from the Family

Psychoeducation is a two-way street. What kinds of questions are most crucial for *you* to ask of family during an inpatient admission? Well, since this is a major crisis, you'll want to focus on immediate triggers and safety concerns.

"It's important that I understand the events leading up to Suzie's admission here. I'd really like to hear your perspective on how things have been going."

Often, the family will give you a very different account from the impression you may have received from interviewing the patient.

CLINICAL VIGNETTE

A 50-year-old woman was admitted after having walked into the emergency room saying that she wanted to die. She said she believed her husband didn't love her anymore and suspected he was seeing another woman. The psychiatrist held a meeting with the husband and the patient's grown daughter the next morning.

Interviewer: Vicki tells me she's been concerned about your relationship.

Husband: (Looking confused). What do you mean "concerned"?

Interviewer: She told me that you have been distant, spending nights out, and maybe seeing someone else.

The husband and the daughter looked bewildered and shook their heads.

Husband: I haven't gone out at night without Vicki since last winter, when I went to a work Christmas party that she didn't want to go to. We're basically joined at the hip.

Interviewer: So what had been happening in the few days before she came to the ER?

Daughter: Mom has been saying strange things. She's been worried about everything. We went to the mall together and she wouldn't go into any of the stores. She said they were dangerous and that there was a "code orange" and there might be terrorists planting bombs in the store.

On further evaluation, it turned out that the patient was suffering a psychotic depression with the paranoid delusion that her husband had been sleeping with a terrorist.

In sum, whether you are evaluating patients in an office setting or in the hospital, do not neglect one of your most valuable resources—the people who know your patients the best.

Techniques for Other Challenging Situations

> **Essential Concepts**
> - The hostile patient
> - The seductive patient
> - The tearful patient

> *Be firm, fair, and understanding. Hold the reins in one hand and a lump of sugar in the other.*
>
> Elvin Semrad
> The Heart of a Therapist

THE HOSTILE PATIENT

When a patient becomes hostile during an initial interview, remember that it's not your fault. Unless you're laughably incompetent or a real creep, a hostile attack is a product of the patient's pathology. Common causes of patient anger during the first meeting include paranoid psychosis, irritability due to depression or mania, and borderline personality disorder. The best way to defuse hostility is to diagnose its cause and then target your intervention accordingly.

The Hostile, Paranoid Patient

The hostile, paranoid patient is angry at you because he perceives you as a direct threat or perhaps as part of an elaborate conspiracy. A good way to counteract this false projection is to use self-effacing humor or general goofiness, which is easier to pull off. The patient usually perceives this attitude as inconsistent with evil intentions.

CLINICAL VIGNETTE

A patient with the diagnosis of bipolar disorder was admitted involuntarily to the inpatient unit because of paranoia concerning her husband, who she believed was trying to have her killed. It was clear from the outset of the interview that she thought that she had been wrongly committed and wanted to leave immediately.

> *Patient: How can you keep me here? You have no right. I can call a lawyer.*
>
> *Interviewer: You can certainly call a lawyer. The reason we...*
>
> *Patient: (Interrupting) I can call a lawyer, but it's not going to do any good, is it? All the lawyers are part of a big game, and they're going to say just what you want them to say.*
>
> *Interviewer: What kind of game do you think this is? Last I checked, this was just a psychiatric hospital.*
>
> *Patient: You know exactly what's going on here, and wipe that innocent look off your face.*
>
> *Interviewer: I'm not innocent. I plead guilty to being a psychiatrist. I'm trying to help you. And if you believe that, I have a bridge in Brooklyn you might be interested in.*
>
> *Patient: What bridge?*
>
> *Interviewer: Oh that's just an old joke, and a bad one. I find that I have to use humor to keep me sane here, you know? But enough about me. What were we talking about?*
>
> *Patient: The people who are trying to have me killed.*

At this point, the patient opened up significantly, and a productive conversation ensued. The attempt at humor was unexpected enough to derail an increasingly hostile train of thought.

The Irritable, Depressed Patient

Depressed patients can come across as hostile, but it is a hostility that cloaks a reservoir of pain. A good technique is to make a fairly direct interpretation, such as

> You sound angry, but I think there's some sadness underneath that anger.
> I can understand how you would be angry with me, but I wonder if there isn't something beneath the anger that's eating at you?

The Patient with Borderline Personality Disorder

Like the irritable, depressed patient, the borderline patient's anger overlies pain. Because of immature coping skills, the patient cannot "sit" with her pain and rationally problem-solve. Instead, she tends to project and externalize, resulting in lashing out that can be quite uncomfortable for you. It isn't easy to maintain your composure during these times, but it helps if you can see the anger as a crisis of aloneness. Be compassionate, and fight against the natural tendency to either fight back or to withdraw into a protective shell of aloofness. Defensiveness will only rile your patient further, and aloofness will deepen her sense of abandonment.

Instead, be curious, interested, and caring. Effective statements for patients with borderline personality disorder often include the following:

> *For the sake of our discussion, what do you think just happened? You're very angry at me, and I'm wondering what that anger is about.*
> *I've done (or said) something that upset you, and I hope to understand what that is so that we can put it behind us and move on with the important work we have to do to help you feel better.*

THE SEDUCTIVE PATIENT

Although seductive behavior often does not become apparent until follow-up sessions, it is helpful to have some idea of how best to respond to overtly seductive behavior. To begin with, renew your own absolute commitment never to become sexually involved with your patients. Aside from breaking professional ethical codes, it is always destructive, to both your patient and yourself. Any practitioner who often finds himself tempted to breach this boundary should obtain therapy or supervision or find another career.

This is not to say that you will never have sexual feelings toward your patients. Of course you will, but if your commitment never to act on such feelings is absolute, you can manage these feelings while continuing to deliver excellent care.

Seductive behavior comes in two guises, subtle and blatant. Subtle behavior includes significant glances, revealing clothes, and excessive curiosity about the interviewer's personal life. Such subtle behavior can be managed in several ways:

- Keep the trappings of the therapeutic relationship relatively formal.
- Use the patient's title and last name.
- Keep the interview focused on the presenting symptoms.
- Avoid small talk.

Deflect requests for personal information with statements such as "The purpose of this interview is for us to get a better understanding of what's been troubling you, and I really think that should be the focus."

Blatant seductive behavior involves more direct questions about the interviewer's availability and requests to be touched or hugged by the therapist or to spend some time outside of the treatment session with her. These behaviors require a direct and unambiguous response that makes it clear that such contact is inappropriate and impossible and explains why. The following vignette illustrates this type of situation.

CLINICAL VIGNETTE

The patient is a woman in her 30s who is in the process of divorcing her husband. She has scheduled a diagnostic interview to evaluate her depression. The interviewer is a married man also in his 30s. The vignette begins toward the end of the interview, and the clinician has already recommended an antidepressant.

> *Interviewer: I also think it would be helpful for you to see a therapist.*
>
> *Patient: Can't you be my therapist?*
>
> *Interviewer: No, I'm a psychopharmacologist, and I schedule brief follow-up visits to check on how well the medication is working.*
>
> *Patient: But I like you.*
>
> *Interviewer: (Beginning to sense a hint of seductiveness) That's good, because I'll continue to monitor your medication, but I think you'd benefit from seeing a therapist for more frequent sessions.*
>
> *Patient: (Smiling seductively) What I'd really like is to meet someone who could be both my therapist and my lover.*

Interviewer: Wait a minute. Let's back up a little. It's very destructive for therapists or psychiatrists to have anything other than a professional relationship with their patients. That will never happen during our treatment, nor will it happen with any therapist you might see. From what you've told me today, I can see you've been feeling lonely, and I think it would be good for you to work on building up friendships, but that will have to happen outside of treatment sessions.

The patient eventually accepted a therapy referral and continued in treatment without overt seductiveness.

THE TEARFUL PATIENT

Many patients cry during the initial appointment, and as a beginning clinician, you may feel at a loss when this happens. You will typically feel your own share of emotions in such situations, which may range from poignant empathy to anxious discomfort. You will probably instinctively want to behave as you would when a close friend or family member cries in front of you, which may include a pat or a hug and comforting words. That is usually a mistake in a professional relationship. So what should you do?

The proper approach will vary from patient to patient. When a patient cries, try to understand the meaning of the tears, which is not always obvious. For example, the patient who cries while describing a recent marital separation may be crying for several reasons, including a feeling of abandonment, a fear of future financial hardship, a sense of personal failure, and a relief that the relationship is over.

When a patient becomes tearful, I recommend offering some tissues, which should always be in your office, waiting empathetically for a few seconds, and then asking any of the following questions:

> *What is it about what you are saying that is so painful?*
> *I can see you're feeling emotional now; what are your tears about?*
> *What's on your mind now as you're crying?*

It's also helpful to ask about the frequency of crying:

Have you been crying a lot about this?

It's quite common for patients to say they have not cried until that very moment, which is usually a validation of your interviewing skills.

If a patient expresses some shame or embarrassment about crying, make a validating statement such as

Crying can be a good release.
Go ahead and cry as much as you need to. It's good that you feel comfortable enough here that you're allowing yourself to cry.
Crying is a big part of the healing process.

Of course, lest I leave you with the impression that crying is a wonderful thing, I should remind you that tears indicate intense emotional pain and should prompt you to be especially vigilant for SI (see Chapter 22).

Practical Psychodynamics in the Diagnostic Interview

> **Essential Concepts**
> - Assess your patient's degree of reality distortion.
> - Detect negative transference and move beyond it.
> - Identify defense mechanisms and coping responses.
> - Use your countertransference diagnostically.

> *It might be said of psychoanalysis that if you give it your little finger it will soon have your whole hand.*
> Sigmund Freud

Keeping an ear open for psychodynamic material can help you in a number of ways as you conduct your diagnostic interviews. First, you can increase the accuracy of your diagnosis, because symptoms are often the product of life circumstances and dysfunctional ways of responding to them. Psychodynamics provides the preeminent language for describing defense mechanisms, and it also helps you understand how to use countertransference toward patients productively. Second, understanding psychodynamic principles will help you manage the interview itself, especially if your patient has negative transference toward you. Finally, understanding defense mechanisms will help you to diagnose personality disorders, which are covered in more detail in Chapter 31.

REALITY DISTORTION

Reality distortion is often the first clue that significant psychodynamic factors may be at work in your patient's psychology. Psychosis is the extreme of reality distortion, but many nonpsychotic patients distort reality as well. Examples include the depressed woman who unfairly castigates herself for being the cause of all misfortune in her family, the narcissist who tells you that all his past therapists have been substandard and therefore unhelpful, and the alcoholic who says her husband is being ridiculous in criticizing her drinking habits.

Often, reality distortions will jump out at you over the course of the interview. Occasionally, you'll need to dig for them. In Chapter 27, I suggest some screening questions to elicit the presence of the delusions. In these patients, however, we're not talking about frank delusions; we're talking about milder distortions. The way to elicit distortions is to be curious about how your patients interpret the motivations of others or how they make sense of events overall.

CLINICAL VIGNETTE

The patient is a 25-year-old woman with a history of panic disorder with agoraphobia and comorbid alcohol abuse. She recently terminated visits to her last psychiatrist because he refused to prescribe benzodiazepines for her anxiety disorder.

> *Patient: Dr. X said, "Absolutely not. I won't give you any Xanax."*
>
> *Interviewer: What do you think was on his mind when he said that? (You are probing for her world view.)*
>
> *Patient: To tell you the truth, I have no idea. Maybe that's his rule.*
>
> *Interviewer: What sort of rule do you mean?*
>
> *Patient: Maybe he never prescribes those kinds of drugs for people like me.*
>
> *Interviewer: People like you?*
>
> *Patient: People with anxiety; people who really need them.*
>
> *Interviewer: Why wouldn't he prescribe meds to people who need them?*
>
> *Patient: Who knows. He's probably burned out. Most shrinks are.*

The patient presents a jaded view of psychiatrists, possibly reflecting a more general view of the world as uncaring. Alternatively, her statements may reflect the defense mechanism of projection, in which the patient disavows her own anger at being deprived of an addictive drug and projects it onto her psychiatrist, who then appears sadistic to her because he doesn't prescribe medications to people who need them. Whatever the nature of her distortions, you can be certain that you will not be exempt from them, and you can begin to prepare your own strategy to prevent future struggles. This might include making statements that demonstrate an understanding of her world view:

> As I listen to you, it sounds like you've gotten the short end of the stick over and over again in life. I wouldn't be surprised if you're assuming that it's going to be the same way here, too.

Once you detect a reality distortion, determine whether defense mechanisms or transference is at work.

NEGATIVE TRANSFERENCE

> Whenever two people meet there are really six people present. There is each man as he sees himself, each man as the other person sees him, and each man as he really is.

> William James

In transference, your patient unconsciously reenacts a past relationship and transfers it to a present relationship; this doesn't necessarily pose a problem in the initial interview. Your patient may have a positive transference toward you, in which you remind him of someone he admired, like his mother, causing him to automatically ascribe to you all kinds of wonderful qualities. Sit back and enjoy it.

Negative transference, however, can be problematic, especially when it involves anger. Your patient may have been poorly treated by people throughout his life, and he expects you to be no different. Look for negative transference when there is a sense of tension. Perhaps your patient is making angry comments or asking provocative questions. Perhaps he is giving monosyllabic answers to your questions.

In psychoanalytic psychotherapy, negative transference is actually elicited, because its interpretation is the backbone of treatment. In the diagnostic interview, however, negative transference is usually counterproductive, and the best way to deal with it is to recognize it and make an empathic comment that neutralizes it. Although there's no easy way of learning how to make these comments—other than practice, practice, and more practice—the following list contains some common statements (in italics) made by patients during diagnostic interviews. Most of these statements reflect negative transference or a defense mechanism of some sort. All of these statements tend to throw novice interviewers for a loop.

Possible hidden meanings are listed after each patient statement; the emphasis is on *possible*. Sometimes, such statements have no hidden meaning and are a statement of fact. For example, you may look bored during an interview and, in fact, feel bored. If the patient is making an accurate observation, don't try to interpret the comment. That is dishonest and unfair to your patient. In addition, the hidden meanings I've listed are illustrative only. They don't imply that all patients making such a statement actually mean what I suggest. You should interpret each statement individually, based on your knowledge of the particular patient.

In general, the possible responses are ways of moving beyond the negative statement, so that the work of the diagnostic interview can proceed. Note that this is a very different approach from what you would do if you were engaged in psychodynamic therapy.

You're not a very helpful doctor.

Possible hidden meaning: *No one has ever cared for me, and you're no exception.*

Possible response (while nodding empathically): "You know, that's not the first time I've heard that, and when I'm not being helpful to a patient I always ask, 'How can I be more helpful? Because I really do want to help.'" (This communicates that you really do care and implies that the therapeutic alliance won't be damaged by your patient's comment, but may actually be strengthened by it.)

Possible hidden meaning: *I'm a very special patient, and you should treat me unusually well.*

Possible response: "I bet it feels disappointing to have a doctor who doesn't come up to snuff. Is it possible, though, that you're judging prematurely?" (Empathize with the patient's injured sense of specialness, while giving him an out to repair the relationship.)

You look bored.

Possible hidden meaning: *Of course you are bored; I'm such a boring person.*

Possible response: "I'm actually not at all bored, but do you think that the things you're saying are boring?"

Possible hidden meaning: I expect you to respond lovingly and immediately to everything I say; if you are silent, I have to assume that you're feeling something negative toward me.

Possible response: "In my profession, silence rarely means boredom. It usually means concentration and interest."

Is that all you're going to do, just sit there silently and nod?

Possible hidden meaning: You're just like my parents, who never expressed any kind of interest in me, who never responded to anything I said.

Possible response: "Does that seem unhelpful? I actually have a lot to say, but I always try to bite my tongue so that my patients get a chance to tell their whole story. I usually find that I'm most helpful to patients only after I've really listened to them and understood them well."

What kind of credentials do you have?

Possible hidden meaning: I'm in a lot of pain, and I'm not certain whether you or anybody else can help me.

Possible response: (Begin by stating your credentials quickly.) "I'm_____ (e.g., an intern, a resident) at_____ (i.e., name of school or hospital). Are you concerned about my ability to help you?"

Possible hidden meaning: I've been made to feel ineffectual all my life, and I want you to get a taste of what that feels like. (This is an example of an immature defense mechanism known as projective identification.)

Possible response: (State your credentials.) "But my main credential is that I'm here with you; I want to understand you and to help you as best I can." (By this, you demonstrate that self-esteem does not depend on getting someone else to say you are effectual.)

You don't show much understanding of what I'm saying.

Possible hidden meaning: I'm angry at you for not understanding me implicitly and fully without my having to be explicit. I want you to be the perfectly empathic parent I never had.

Possible response: "You know, I couldn't agree more. It is so hard for one person to really understand another person. But why don't we talk some more, and I'll give it my best shot."

Are you married?

Possible hidden meaning: I wish I were married to you.

Another possible hidden meaning: I'll bet you are married, and that you have a wonderful spouse, proving how much better you are than I am and what a loser I am.

Possible response (with a smile): "Wait a minute! I thought I was the one who's supposed to be asking the questions here."

Another possible response: "You know what? I've found that when I start answering questions about my personal life, it can get in the way of my understanding you better, and isn't that the whole point of our hour together?"

DEFENSE MECHANISMS AND COPING RESPONSES

When uncomfortable and unpleasant emotions arise, we all have ways of lessening the brunt of them. We use defense mechanisms. The classifications in Table 13.1 are adapted from Vaillant's (1988) hierarchy of defense mechanisms.

TABLE 13.1. Classification of Defense Mechanisms

Mature defenses
  Suppression
  Altruism
  Sublimation
  Humor
Neurotic defenses
  Denial
  Repression
  Reaction formation
  Displacement
  Rationalization
Immature defenses
  Passive aggression
  Acting out
  Dissociation
  Projection
  Splitting (idealization/devaluation)
Psychotic defenses
  Denial of external reality
  Distortion of external reality

Adapted from Vaillant, G. E. (1988). Defense mechanisms. In A. M. Nicholi, Jr. (Ed.), *The New Harvard Guide to Psychiatry* (p. 81). Cambridge, MA: Harvard University Press.

Main Defense Mechanisms

Following are brief definitions and examples of the different defense mechanisms. The examples included here are various ways that a patient might react if, in this instance, her husband left her.

Mature Defenses

Mature defenses usually arise from, and lead to, psychological health rather than from dysfunction.

Suppression

- Definition: Emotion remains conscious but is suppressed.
- Example: I'm disappointed and sad, but I won't let these emotions interfere significantly with my life.

Altruism

- Definition: Suppressing the emotion by doing something nice for others.
- Example: I'll volunteer at a women's shelter.

Sublimation

- Definition: Transmuting the emotion into a productive and socially redeeming endeavor.
- Example: I'll start immediately on a book about how to cope with rejection.

Humor

- Definition: Expressing the emotion in an indirect and humorous way.
- Example: This is great! I've been trying for years to get rid of 180 pounds of ugly fat.

Neurotic (Transitional) Defenses

Neurotic defenses are less healthy than mature defenses because they tend to cause psychological distress either immediately, as with repression or displacement, or in the future, when the actual pain eventually surfaces.

Denial

- Definition: Denying that the emotion exists.
- Example: The rejection doesn't bother me at all.

Repression

- Definition: Stuffing the emotion out of conscious awareness. (Unfortunately, the emotion typically returns to haunt the repressor in unpredictable ways.)
- Example: I didn't feel at all bad about his leaving me, but for the past few weeks, I've had this splitting headache, and I don't know why.

Reaction Formation

- Definition: Forgetting the negative emotion by transforming it into its opposite.
- Example: We've become such close friends since this happened. He is really a wonderful person.

Displacement

- Definition: Displacing the emotion from its original object to something or someone else.
- Example: My boss has really been getting under my skin lately.

Rationalization

- Definition: Inventing a convincing, but usually false, reason why you are *not* bothered.
- Example: I've been wanting to make some major life changes anyway. This finally gave me the boost I needed to do all the things I've been wanting to do.

Immature Defenses

Immature defenses lead to more severe distress and often have a negative impact on other people.

Passive Aggression

- Definition: Expressing anger indirectly and passively.
- Example: Oh, I'm sorry, dear. I gave all your clothes to the Salvation Army last week. I didn't realize you wanted them.

Acting Out

- Definition: Expressing the emotion in actions rather than keeping it in awareness.
- Example: (The patient makes harassing, late-night phone calls.)

Dissociation

- Definition: Dissociating instead of feeling the pain.
- Example: I was really spaced out all of last week; my memory of him leaving me is very hazy.

Projection

- Definition: Disavowing the anger and ascribing it to the object of the anger.
- Example: I'm convinced that ever since he left me, he's been bad-mouthing me to all our friends.

Splitting (Idealization/Devaluation)

- Definition: Defining the rejecting person as being all bad versus having seen him as all good before the rejection, thereby transforming pain into anger and accusation.
- Example: I always knew he was a horrible person, and this proves it. May he rot in hell.

Psychotic Defenses

Psychotic defenses so completely flaunt external reality that they signal a psychotic thought process (TP).

Denial of External Reality

- Definition is self-explanatory.
- Example: He never left me.

Distortion of External Reality

- Definition is self-explanatory.
- Example: He didn't leave me! He went off on a business trip. He'll be back next week.

In the diagnostic interview, identifying defense mechanisms is useful to quickly sense whether your patient may have a personality disorder (such patients typically use immature defenses) and to give you a sense of prognosis (patients who use higher level defenses tend to do better than others).

As you listen to your patient with a psychodynamic ear, ask yourself the following questions:

- How does the patient seem to shelter himself from the psychological pain that he is sharing with you?
- Does he tend to use mature or immature defenses?
- Do his defenses tend to bring him out of his misery (mature defenses) or steep him more deeply in it (neurotic and immature defenses)?
- If you were his therapist, which of his defenses would you encourage and which would you point out to him as unproductive?

At the end of the interview, before you write up the evaluation, you'll find it helpful to review the defenses (see the pocket cards in Appendix A) and determine which one(s) the patient seems to use. Make a habit of spending at least a few moments thinking about the defenses your patients use. This will help you to better recognize defenses in the future.

COPING STYLES

Coping styles and defense mechanisms are similar concepts. Vaillant (1988) distinguishes coping responses from defense mechanisms: Coping, he says, "involves eliciting help from appropriate others" and "voluntary cognitive efforts like information gathering, anticipating danger, and rehearsing responses to danger" (Vaillant 1988, p. 200). Defense mechanisms, on the other hand, are *involuntary* cognitive responses to stressors that usually fit into one of the categories listed in the prior section.

Think of coping as a series of active behavioral and cognitive responses designed to overcome a stressful event. You will typically be able to evaluate your patient's coping styles by listening to her HPI and hearing how she dealt with the distress. It is not surprising that the coping responses of many psychiatric patients are not very effective.

How did your patient respond to the main problems described in the HPI? If depression is the problem, did he cope adaptively, by, for example, contacting friends or family for support; decreasing his responsibilities for a while; or doing something that he knew would give him pleasure, such as seeing a movie or going on a vacation? Or did he cope maladaptively, by isolating himself, by lashing out at people close to him, or through self-mutilating behavior?

If anxiety is a major problem, did he use positive coping strategies, such as telling himself the anxiety will pass, taking deep breaths, taking a walk? Or did he use more negative strategies, such as visiting hospital emergency rooms excessively, using alcohol or other drugs, or bingeing on sweets?

As with defense mechanisms, seek to encourage positive coping responses and to discourage negative ones.

USING COUNTERTRANSFERENCE DIAGNOSTICALLY

Countertransference refers to the whole range of emotions that you may feel toward your patient, whether positive or negative. Novice interviewers have a tendency to try to suppress or ignore such feelings, especially when they are negative. Don't. These countertransference feelings represent some of the most clinically valuable material available to you. Whatever feelings your patient elicits in you are feelings she probably elicits in most other people she encounters in her life. Knowing this can give you powerful insight into the nature of her problems.

CLINICAL VIGNETTE

A 45-year-old man was admitted to the psychiatric unit for depression and suicidal ideation (SI). He had recently been fired from his job, and he complained of loneliness, as he had lost most of his friends over the years. I did the admission interview, and the following exchange occurred 5 minutes into it.

> *Interviewer: How long had you been feeling depressed?*
> *Patient: Quite a while. But tell me, aren't you just a resident?*
> *Interviewer: (Immediately feeling defensive.) Well, yes, I'm the chief resident of the unit.*
> *Patient: (He narrows his eyes.) Chief resident. I see. That's a pretty political position, isn't it?*

Interviewer: (*Increasingly uncomfortable and caught off guard.*) *No, I wouldn't say it's a particularly political position. I supervise the other residents.*

Patient: *Yes, but there's always someone watching over you, isn't there? If you do well, maybe you'll get a nice job in the department. I know how it works. I'd prefer to talk to a full attending, someone who isn't always looking over his shoulder.*

Interviewer: (*Feeling enraged and suppressing the urge to scream at him and kick him out of the office.*) *In fact, you will be talking to an attending in the morning, but I do need to talk to you briefly this afternoon.*

The patient agreed to proceed with the interview and answered questions briefly and disdainfully. On further assessment, a picture of severe narcissistic personality disorder emerged, and my countertransference reaction made it graphically understandable how he had managed to alienate all the important people in his life, leading to his current depression.

The bottom line is that when you feel a negative emotion toward your patient, don't act on it. Instead, analyze its possible connection to your patient's psychopathology.

II

THE PSYCHIATRIC
HISTORY

Obtaining the History
of Present Illness

WHAT IS THE HISTORY OF PRESENT ILLNESS?

The HPI is probably the most important part of the psychiatric interview, and yet, there is disagreement on exactly what it should entail. Even experienced clinicians differ in how they approach the HPI. Some think of it as the "history of present crisis" and focus on the preceding few weeks. Such clinicians begin their interviews with questions such as, "What has been going on recently that brings you into the clinic today?" Others begin by eliciting the entire history of the patient's primary syndrome: "Tell me about your depression. How old were you when you first felt depressed?" These clinicians work forward to the present episode.

Each of these approaches may be useful, depending on the clinical situation. If a patient has a relatively uncomplicated and brief psychiatric history, it might make sense to explore that first and then move to the HPI. If the psychiatric history is long, with many hospitalizations and caregivers, starting at the beginning may bring you too far from the present problem.

The most common pitfall for beginners is spending too much time on the HPI. It's easy to do, because this is the time for your patient to share the most difficult and painful part of his story, and cutting your patient off as time begins to pass may seem unempathic. Thus, it is vital that you keep in mind the advice offered in Section I about asking questions and changing topics sensitively. Use these techniques to gently but persistently bring the patient back to the HPI.

In the following sections, I describe techniques for the two major approaches to the HPI; you should decide which to use for a given patient.

The History of Present Crisis Approach

The *American Heritage Dictionary* defines *crisis* as "A crucial point or situation in the course of anything; a turning point." As you begin the interview, ask yourself, "Why now? Why is this a crucial point in this person's life? What has been happening recently to bring her into my office?" Often, psychiatric crises occur over a 1- to 4-week period, so focus your initial questions on this period.

> *What has been happening over the past week or two that has brought you into the clinic?*
> *Tell me about some of the stressors you've dealt with over the past couple of weeks.*

History of the Syndrome Approach

Alternatively, you can begin your questioning by ascertaining when the patient first remembers signs of the illness.

> *When did you first begin having these kinds of problems?*
> *When was the last time you remember feeling perfectly well?*

Ensuing questions track the course of the illness through months or years, arriving eventually at the present.

> *Now let's talk about this current episode. When did it start?*

One nice thing about this approach to the HPI is that most case write-ups are organized in this format—they often begin, "The patient was without any psychiatric problems until age 18, when she became depressed...."

TIP: MAKING THE INTERVIEW ELEGANT, OR THE "BARBARA WALTERS APPROACH"

At its best, a well-conducted interview resembles a dance in which the give and take between clinician and patient flow effortlessly throughout the hour, giving the patient the sense that he just participated in a fascinating conversation about his life rather than a "psychiatric" interview. One way to set the stage for this type of experience is to begin the interview by showing genuine interest and curiosity about the patient's job, hobbies, or life situation and to allow the patient to steer the discussion toward clinical topics. Imagine that you are Barbara Walters interviewing a celebrity, bringing that same intense curiosity to your patient:

> **Interviewer:** *I see from your intake sheet that you work for the IRS. What do you do with them?*
> **Patient:** *I'm in their call center, but it's only seasonal.*
> **Interviewer:** *So when I call the IRS to ask for a form, you might answer?*
> **Patient:** *Yes, but I do a lot more. I can answer questions about a customer's return.*
> **Interviewer:** *Wait, you're kidding. If I were to call you and ask how much I owed, you'd be able to pull that information up while I was on the phone.*
> **Patient:** *Oh yes, we have the whole database available, at least when the computers aren't down! It's really a great job, my first good job, but during the summer I'm usually laid off, and I don't know why (patient appears dejected).*
> **Interviewer:** *That's too bad, why do they lay you off? (The patient begins to describe difficulties leading up to her current depression.)*

ELICIT A CHRONOLOGIC NARRATIVE, EMPHASIZING PRECIPITANTS

Many patients automatically jump into a chronologic narrative of their problems when prompted by one of the preceding questions. If this happens, it is a time to fall silent for a while and listen. Remember, this is your "scouting period" (see Chapter 3), during which you are observing, listening, and hypothesizing. However, if your patient begins to jump around into other issues or time frames, you may want to refocus him.

> *Patient: I felt so angry when my wife yelled at me. But she's always been that way. Back when I was in law school, she nagged at me constantly. I'd have to spend late nights at the law library, and she refused to understand.*
>
> *Interviewer: I'd like to hear more about that period later, but right now let's focus on what's been happening over the last 2 weeks or so. You said you got angry at her. What happened then?*

Ask the patient specifically about potential precipitants for her suffering:

> *Have there been any events that have caused your problem or made it worse?*

Occasionally, the patient will deny any precipitants. This is particularly true of patients who view their psychiatric illness from a medical model. Such a patient might answer the question above with

> *No, I can't think of anything that's causing it. My life is going pretty well; I just keep getting these depressions.*

Certainly, some psychiatric illnesses, such as bipolar disorder, can have lives of their own, but it's unusual for patients to decompensate without some precipitant. Often, patients haven't associated particular events with their pain and simply need their memories jogged. Make it a practice to dig by asking about specific events that commonly destabilize patients (Table 14.1). You won't necessarily ask about every item on this list, of course. You may already have some clues

TABLE 14.1. Common Precipitants of Psychiatric Syndromes

Arguments with friends or relatives
Rejection or abandonment
Death or major illness of loved one
Anniversary of a negative event, such as a death or divorce
Major medical illness or age-related deterioration in functioning
Stressful events at work or school
Mental health clinician going on vacation
Medication noncompliance
Substance abuse

from an earlier part of the interview that one of these events is particularly likely. As you ask these questions, remember that correlation does not equal causality. A stressful psychosocial event may have occurred around the time of a psychiatric problem and yet be unrelated to it.

LAUNCH INTO THE DIAGNOSTIC QUESTIONS RIGHT AWAY

One of the secrets of efficient and rapid diagnostic interviewing is a gentle tenacity; when the patient mentions a depressed mood, immediately assess for the presence of the diagnostic criteria for depression.

> *Patient: I think the worst problem over the past couple of weeks is that I've felt so down about myself.*
> *Interviewer: Has that down feeling been affecting your sleep?*
> *Patient: I haven't slept more than 2 or 3 hours a night, and the next day, I can barely drag myself to work. I should probably quit anyway; it's a boring job.*
> *Interviewer: Have you had problems focusing on your work because of your depression?*

Here, the interviewer stays on the depression topic by cueing off what the patient has said about work (see the discussion of the smooth transition in Chapter 6). If the interviewer had not actively structured the interview this way, the patient might have discussed details of his work environment that would be less relevant to the diagnosis of major depression. Later, when ascertaining the social history, the interviewer can refer to what the patient said about work:

> *Interviewer: Earlier, you mentioned that your work is boring. How did you get into that line of work? (Note the use of the referred transition.)*

CURRENT AND PREMORBID LEVEL OF FUNCTIONING

The now outdated *DSM-IV-TR* diagnostic scheme included an "Axis V" in which you noted the patient's "GAF," or global assessment of functioning, on a scale of 0 to 100. Although

I never found it useful to assign a specific number to functioning (only insurance companies were obsessed with that number), I do think that Axis V was an important reminder to the interviewer to ask about both current and baseline functioning.

To assess overall functioning, ask about the three basic aspects of life: love, work, and fun. Love includes all important relationships: family, spouse, and close friends. In addition to paid employment, *work* includes school, volunteer activities, and the structured day activities in which many chronically mentally ill patients participate. *Fun* refers to hobbies and recreational pursuits.

> *How has your illness been affecting your work, relationships, and leisure pursuits?*

The phrasing of this question automatically targets the patient's premorbid functioning. Some patients have a hard time distinguishing a psychiatric illness from the rest of their lives. If so, you will have to follow up with another question to assess their baseline functioning.

> *Before you started to have these anxiety spells (or other symptoms), how was work going?*
> *How were you getting along with your family and your wife?*
> *What kinds of things were you doing for fun?*

For patients who have more chronic illnesses with multiple exacerbations and remissions, ask the same types of questions about periods between exacerbations:

> *Think about the last time that you were feeling your best, when you weren't hearing any voices and you didn't feel suicidal. How was your life going then? (Follow up with questions about love, work, and fun.)*

Asking about current versus baseline functioning is important diagnostically. The classic example is the difference between schizophrenia and bipolar disorder. In schizophrenia, the patient's level of functioning gradually decreases over months or years, whereas in bipolar disorder, the patient may have been functioning dramatically better within the past few weeks. Determining baseline functioning is also important in setting treatment goals. You might aim to help the patient achieve his best level of functioning over the past year, for example.

CLINICAL VIGNETTE

A resident was working in a busy psychiatric crisis clinic and interviewed a patient who was brought by ambulance for psychotic and disorganized behavior. The patient was a 32-year-old woman and carried the diagnosis of "schizoaffective disorder" in her previous emergency department records. The phrase "history of multiple psychiatric hospitalizations" in the old chart caused the resident to assume that the patient was a chronically poorly functioning woman who could rarely stay out of a hospital. In assessing her psychosocial functioning, the resident was surprised to learn that the patient had been working as a secretary for a research department of a local hospital until 1 year ago, when she had the first of a series of recent hospitalizations. This information caused the resident to pay closer attention to the patient's history and to entertain the possibility of a different diagnosis, such as borderline personality disorder or PTSD, both of which would be more consistent with her good premorbid functioning.

Obtaining the
Psychiatric History

The past psychiatric history (PPH) risks becoming a tedious exercise in documentation. You can avoid this by realizing how vital the PPH is to your twin goals of establishing a diagnosis and formulating a treatment plan.

Specific psychiatric disorders have specific natural histories, with characteristic risk factors, prodromal signs, ages at onset, and prognoses. Obtaining a detailed PPH for a particular patient allows you to compare the course of *her* illness with the textbook's version of the course of illness, increasing the likelihood that you will make a correct diagnosis.

Often, patients will come to you after having been treated for many years. One reason such patients are eventually referred to an expert consultant is that experts are great at eliciting a *detailed history of prior treatments*. They can determine exactly what has been tried in the past and whether past treatment trials have been adequate. From this information, they can present informed recommendations about what should be tried next. *And* they can do all this in one or two 50-minute sessions.

Potential pitfalls in obtaining the PPH are similar to those lurking during the HPI. At one end of the continuum, some interviewers become so caught up in the intricacies of the PPH that they spend most of the evaluation time on it, to the detriment of, for example, the PROS. At the other end, the PPH can become a rote exercise and may be obtained too superficially, depriving the interviewer of information necessary to make a firm diagnosis.

OBTAIN THE SYNDROMAL HISTORY

Generally speaking, the HPI will take between 5 and 10 minutes, at the end of which you should have a few provisional diagnoses in mind. Your next job is to obtain the history of these syndromes. Specifically, you want to learn age at onset, premorbid functioning, and history of subsequent episodes up to the present.

Age at Onset

> *How old were you when you first had your symptoms?*

Knowing the age at onset may help you to decide between potential diagnoses, with anxiety disorders having a much earlier onset than either mood disorders or schizophrenia (Jones 2013).

Premorbid Functioning or Baseline Functioning

See Chapter 14 for a discussion of premorbid functioning/ baseline functioning.

History and Precipitants of Subsequent Episodes up to Present

Include questions about the severity of episodes and exacerbations, as well as the duration of episodes. Often, this information comes out when you are obtaining the treatment history. For example, episodes of mania or exacerbations of schizophrenia often correspond with hospitalizations.

As with hospitalizations, a time-efficient method of asking about episodes is to ask about the first one, the latest one, and the total number of episodes.

- When did you have your first breakdown?
- How many have you had in total?
- When was your last one?

OBTAIN THE TREATMENT HISTORY

You ask about prior treatments mostly to help with future treatment decisions but also to help nail down a diagnosis. For example, if lithium was helpful for an affective episode, bipolar disorder would be high on your list. You want to know what has been tried in the past and whether it has worked. Accuracy and detail are important here, because a sloppy treatment history can lead to poor future treatment decisions. For example, patients may be falsely labeled "treatment resistant" on the basis of old records indicating that numerous medications were "tried but were unsuccessful." On closer questioning, such patients may in fact have had few adequate trials of medication.

I suggest the following format for obtaining the treatment history:

> General questions
> Current caregivers
> Hospitalization history
> Medication history
> Psychotherapy history

Use the mnemonic **Go CHaMP** so that you don't miss any category.

You won't necessarily ask your questions in the above order—in fact, you will obtain much of this information during the HPI—but it's helpful to think about these five aspects of the treatment history to make sure that you haven't neglected to ask important questions. At some point during the interview, mentally review whether you have obtained enough information about each of these categories.

General Questions

> *What sort of treatment have you had for your depression?*
> *What was the most helpful?*

More sophisticated and forthcoming patients will tell you almost everything you need to know about the treatment history in response to a general question. Other patients will require more specific questioning.

> *What was going on in your life during the period when you were depression free?*

In some cases, the best "treatment" for a particular patient was a close relationship with someone or their escape from a dysfunctional relationship. You can learn this from a careful history, and it may become a part of your treatment recommendations.

Current Caregivers

You will need to know who your patient is seeing currently. If he is a new patient, you may be the only caregiver. If you are interviewing a patient with a chronic mental illness, he will likely have both a therapist and a psychopharmacologist, and he may also have a case worker (usually a social worker), a group therapist, and a primary care doctor (a family practitioner or an internist) and may be involved in day treatment or residential treatment.

Hospitalization History

> *Have you ever been hospitalized for a psychiatric problem?*

For patients who have had multiple hospitalizations, do not spend your time ascertaining the names of the hospitals and dates of each admission; this could take the entire 50 minutes. Instead, find out when they were first and last hospitalized and about how many hospitalizations they've had over their lifetime. If a patient has had many hospitalizations, try to find out if they are clustered around a specific few years. Some patients will have had several hospitalizations earlier in the course of their disorder because they had little insight into their problem and were noncompliant with their medications. Later in life, their hospitalizations may be spaced much farther apart. Alternatively, the opposite pattern may appear, in which an affective disorder worsens with age. Think of hospitalizations as markers of disease severity.

> *When were you first hospitalized?*
> *How many hospitalizations have you had in your life?*
> *How many have you had in the past year?*
> *When was your last hospitalization?*

In addition to asking these questions, it is often useful to ask why your patient was hospitalized:

> *In general, what sorts of things have caused you to need to be in the hospital?*

Your assumptions about reason for hospitalization may be wrong, as illustrated by the following example.

CLINICAL VIGNETTE

A patient with chronic schizophrenia stated that he'd been hospitalized several times over the past 2 years. The resident initially assumed that these hospitalizations were for psychotic decompensations, but when asked, the patient said that most were alcohol detoxification admissions. This prompted the resident to obtain a much more thorough substance abuse history than he had planned.

Medication History

> *The most important limit on the bioavailability of medication has nothing to do with pharmacodynamics or pharmacokinetics; rather, it is patient noncompliance.*
>
> Dr. Ross Baldessarini
> Chief of Psychopharmacology
> McLean Hospital

> *Have you been on medications for your depression?*

To the extent possible, document all the medications the patient has tried. Many patients will not remember generic names or may only remember what the pill looked like or the side effect it caused. Obviously, the more you know about alternative names, shapes, and side effects of medication, the more efficiently you will be able to obtain this history. I find smartphone apps such as Epocrates to be helpful, because they have photographs of medications, which help patients identify them. For psychologists and social workers, a number of books have been published that teach the basics of psychopharmacology to non-MDs, and I recommend that you become familiar with this information.

For how many weeks did you take your medications?

Many psychiatric medications take several weeks to have a therapeutic effect. Antidepressants take 4 to 6 weeks. Antipsychotics may take 1 to 2 weeks or longer, depending on the clinical situation. Thus, merely documenting that a patient has tried a particular medication does not mean that he's had an *adequate* trial.

At this point, a normalizing question may be helpful:

> *Often, people do not necessarily take their medications every day but will take them every so often, depending on how they feel. Was that true for you?*

 TIP: HOW ACCURATE ARE PATIENTS WHEN RECALLING PRIOR TREATMENTS?

A fascinating study examined this clinically relevant but under-explored question (Posternak and Zimmerman 2003). An independent evaluator interviewed 73 patients who had been treated in an academic psychiatric clinic for an average of 3.5 years. After the interview, researchers reviewed clinic charts to determine how accurately the patients recalled their antidepressant trials. The results? They did pretty well, overall, recalling 80% of the monotherapy (single medication) trials over the prior 5 years. However, they only remembered 26% of augmentation trials (i.e., when a second medication is added to the first to boost the response). And augmentation trials that were over 2 years old were not remembered by *anybody*. The bottom line is that your patient will accurately recall medications tried if the regimen has always been simple, but those who have taken combinations of medications will be much less reliable.

CLINICAL VIGNETTE

A resident was doing a psychopharmacologic evaluation of a 46-year-old married Latino woman with a several-year history of depression and anxiety. During the treatment history, the patient stated that she had taken a number of different antidepressants from different classes with only minimal effectiveness. The resident asked a normalizing question about whether the patient had taken her medications consistently; she responded that she only took them when she felt anxious, which varied from daily to once every 2 weeks. In fact, the resident was unable to document an adequate trial of *any* antidepressant and subsequently focused on educating the patient on the necessity of consistently taking medications.

Psychotherapy History

In recent years, psychotherapies have become increasingly tailored to specific disorders, and evidence of effectiveness has become irrefutable (Barlow 2014). In addition, it has become clear that therapy can have negative side effects, as can medication. Thus, obtaining a history of psychotherapeutic treatments is important.

> *Have you ever had counseling or therapy for your problem?*
> *How often did you see your therapist?*
> *How long did you see him/her?*

These basic parameters of session frequency and length of treatment are usually nonthreatening and easy to elicit.

> *What sort of therapy did you have?*
> *Did it have a name, like "cognitive therapy," "behavior therapy," or "psychodynamic therapy"?*

More often than not, your patient will not know the technical name of the therapy he received. You can compensate for this by describing the therapy.

> *Did your therapist focus on "automatic thoughts" that make you more anxious or depressed?*
> *Did she give you homework assignments between sessions?*

> *Did she have you practice doing things that caused you anxiety? (For cognitive-behavioral therapy.)*
> *Did your therapist focus on your childhood experiences and how those affect your current life? (For psychodynamic therapy.)*

You can also ask a more open-ended question:

> *Without going into too much detail, what sorts of things did you focus on in therapy?*
> *Was your therapist a psychologist, a psychiatrist, or a social worker?*

Knowing this may or may not be useful. For example, a patient may say she had a therapist, when in fact she was seen by a psychiatrist once a month for brief visits. This was more likely psychopharmacologic management than psychotherapy.

> *How did you like working with your therapist?*
> *Was the therapy helpful?*
> *In what ways was it helpful?*

This information will be particularly valuable in assessing the patient's suitability for further therapy.

> *How did you leave treatment?*

The way a patient ended treatment may tell you much about how he viewed treatment and may help you plan how to proceed with your own treatment of the patient. Some patients, for instance, have a history of ending therapy by simply not showing up for the next session. Others may have had a stormy termination. Others may have terminated "by the book" but continue to feel unexpressed sad or angry feelings toward the therapist.

Screening for General Medical Conditions

There are two major reasons for asking about the medical history in psychiatric patients:

- **To screen for medical illnesses.** Many psychiatric patients, particularly patients with chronic schizophrenia in public care systems, have very poor medical follow-up, both because they are indigent and because their psychiatric disorder leads to poor compliance with appointments (Hall et al. 1980). Thus, they may have a high prevalence of undiagnosed medical conditions. Whether these conditions affect their psychiatric status or not, you will do them a large service by screening for medical conditions for which they may not be receiving treatment.
- **To uncover general medical causes of psychiatric illness.** A number of medical illnesses and medications can cause psychiatric syndromes and aggravate preexisting ones (David and Fleminger 2012). This is a convenient section of the interview for asking about such illnesses.

MIDAS

If you can develop the **MIDAS** touch, you'll never forget to ask about the medical history:

Medications
Illness history
Primary care Doctor
Allergies
Surgical history

Medications

Obtain a list of all medications, including those for general medical conditions. Ascertain whether the patient has been taking them as prescribed.

History of Medical Illnesses

You can begin with a screening question such as

Do you have any medical problems?
Have you ever had a medical illness?

However, a common problem with this approach occurs when the patient says "no" without thinking carefully, as the following vignette illustrates.

CLINICAL VIGNETTE

A 36-year-old woman with several past hospitalizations for depression was asked if she had any medical problems, to which she replied, "No." Later, when the resident asked what medications she took, she listed a number of psychotropics and then said, "and I also take Synthroid." The resident said, "I thought you had no medical problems," to which the patient replied, "I don't. I used to have hypothyroidism, but that was corrected with the Synthroid."

Primary Care Doctor

In the preceding vignette, asking about illness elicited invalid information. One way to increase the validity of your medical history questions is to first ask if the patient is being seen by a doctor.

> *Do you see a doctor regularly?*
> *What does he/she treat you for?*

By referring to a relationship with a caregiver, you will typically jog the patient's memory for past diagnoses and treatments. You can also learn information about the patient's character:

> *Interviewer: Do you see a doctor regularly?*
> *Patient: Yeah, I see someone at the clinic. Not that he gives a damn about me.*

Such a statement could be explored further and might be a clue to character traits that may interfere with treatment, such as passive-aggressive or self-defeating traits.

While you're at it, ask the patient if you may contact his doctor to share information. Discussing the patient with the primary care physician will help round out your evaluation, as well as provide useful information to the caregiver who referred the patient to you.

Allergies

The usual screening question is

> *Do you have allergies to any medications?*

This may work, but again there are potential pitfalls. Some patients have idiosyncratic understandings of what constitutes an allergy. They may think you're asking about serious allergic reactions, such as bronchospasm, and therefore may answer in the negative even if they've had milder allergic reactions. They also may not realize that you're interested in hearing about any negative reactions to medications, and not just allergies per se. Better to ask

> *Have you ever had any allergies, reactions, or side effects to any medication?*

A patient may say that he is allergic to a number of medications that only uncommonly produce true allergic reactions, such as neuroleptics and antidepressants. If so, pursue the nature of the allergy.

> *What kinds of reactions did you have to that medicine?*

If the patient's response is vague, make some suggestions based on your knowledge of drug effects:

> *Did the Haldol give you muscle spasms? Did it make your hands shake or your body move slowly?*

When you document allergies in your write-up, specify the nature of the reaction. For example, writing that a patient is "allergic to neuroleptics" is probably inaccurate and might mean that the patient will never again be offered a neuroleptic, even if she could benefit from it. A more accurate statement would be, "Haldol causes dystonia." This leaves the door open to trials of other neuroleptics.

Surgical History

It is important to ask specifically about previous surgery; many patients do not volunteer this information when asked about "medical problems," either because it was too long ago or because they do not consider an operation to have indicated a medical problem per se.

CLINICAL VIGNETTE

A 54-year-old man with major depression had mentioned gastritis as his only medical problem. Midway through the interview, he mentioned in passing, "I divorced my wife back in '84 or so, just after they took out part of my pancreas." On further exploration, the patient considered that operation to be a turning point in his life, because he made the decision to stop drinking then and had been sober since.

MEDICAL REVIEW OF SYSTEMS

The purpose of the review of symptoms is to note medical problems that the patient may have forgotten to describe in response to the MIDAS questions. Whether it's necessary to do a review of symptoms for every patient is a matter of controversy. The MIDAS questions may miss seemingly minor symptoms that may be the first clues to a big problem,

TABLE 16.1. Brief Versus Full Review of Symptoms

Review of Symptoms	Patient	Rationale
Brief	Young; middle or upper class	Statistically, fewer medical problems; good follow-up with doctors
Full	Elderly; chronically mentally ill	Statistically, more medical problems; poor follow-up with doctors

such as the occasional cough that signals lung cancer. But the review of symptoms takes a lot of time, and most mental health clinicians refer their patients to an internist for physical examinations anyway.

Here's a compromise. I'll outline two approaches to the review of symptoms, a brief review of symptoms (1 minute) and a more extended one (5 minutes) (Table 16.1). Which approach is better depends on the patient and the clinical setting.

Both the brief and extended reviews of symptoms begin with systemic questions and progress in head-to-toe order, which is an easy way to remember them and to ensure that you do not forget to ask important questions.

Brief Review of Systems

I'm going to ask whether you're having problems with various parts of your body, moving from your head to your toes. Any problems with headaches or seizures? Vision or hearing problems? Smelling, taste, or throat problems? Thyroid problems? Problems with your lungs like pneumonia or coughing? Heart problems? Stomach problems like ulcers or constipation? Problems with urination? Joint problems? Problems walking?

Extended Review of Systems
General

Overall, do you feel healthy?
Do you have joint problems or skin problems? (May indicate systemic lupus.)
Do you have excessive bleeding or anemia? (Anemia can cause depression.)

Do you have diabetes or thyroid problems? (Diabetes can cause lethargy; thyroid problems can cause depression or mania.)
Have you ever had cancer?
Do you have any infections, such as HIV or tuberculosis (TB)? (HIV can mimic many psychiatric disorders; TB can mimic depression.)

HEENT (Head, Eyes, Ears, Nose, and Throat)

Do you get headaches? (Can be caused by brain tumor.)
Have you ever had a head injury? (Can lead to neuro-psychiatric conditions.)
Any problems with your vision or your hearing?
Do you ever see or hear things that other people don't notice? (Provides a convenient place to ask about psychotic phenomena in a nonthreatening way.)
Do you get nosebleeds?
Do you smell things that other people don't? (Often a sign of temporal lobe epilepsy.)
How are your teeth?
Do you often get sore throats?

Cardiovascular and Respiratory

Do you have any heart problems?
Do you have chest pains; do you have palpitations of your heart?
Do you have high blood pressure?
Do you experience shortness of breath (emphysema, coronary artery disease)?
Do you cough excessively (lung cancer)?
Do you wheeze (asthma)?

NOTES

Differentiate panic attack from cardiac disease; rule out congestive heart failure as a cause of lethargy and fatigue that might be mistakenly diagnosed as depression. Look for diagnostic clues to the presence of lung cancer, which can mimic the anorexia and weight loss of depression.

Gastrointestinal

> *Do you have problems with nausea or vomiting?*
> *Do you ever make yourself vomit? (A screen for bulimic behavior.)*
> *Do you have problems swallowing?*
> *Do you have constipation or diarrhea?*
> *Have you noticed any change in your stool?*

NOTES

Rule out hidden colon or stomach cancer; diagnose irritable bowel syndrome, which often accompanies psychiatric complaints. Answers to these questions may provide direction in the choice of medications (e.g., you'd want to avoid a tricyclic antidepressant in a patient with preexisting constipation).

Genitourinary and Gynecologic

> *Do you have problems with urination, such as burning or excessive urination?*
> *Do you have retention of urine or incontinence?*
> *Do you have any problems with sexual functioning or sexual drive?*
> *Have you ever had a venereal disease (HIV, syphilis)?*
> *When were your last Pap smear and mammogram?*
> *Do you have any problems with menstruation? When was your last menstrual period?*
> *Might you be pregnant?*

NOTES

Rule out bladder cancer; prostate cancer in men; and uterine, ovarian, or breast cancer in women. Establish amenorrhea of anorexia nervosa. Determine contraindications to the use of anticholinergic medications, such as an enlarged prostate.

Neurologic

> *Have you had seizures?*
> *Have you ever passed out?*
> *Have you ever had a stroke?*
> *Any tingling in your arms or legs?*
> *Any problems with walking, coordination, and balance?*
> *Any problems talking or thinking?*
> *Any changes in your handwriting?*

NOTES

Detect brain tumor, epilepsy, and stroke. Screen for multiple sclerosis, Parkinson's disease, and dementia.

Assessing HIV Risk[1]

I've set up a separate category for HIV risk because it's particularly important, and it can be an awkward subject to bring up. Later in the interview, during the social history, you'll ask some questions about intimate relationships to assess your patient's capacity for relatedness. Here, you focus on sexual functioning as it relates to risk of HIV, but this may lead to a discussion of other concerns.

Begin with an introductory statement such as

> *Here are some questions I routinely ask. Some may be uncomfortable; let me know if they are.*
> *If I may, I'd like to ask you some sexual history questions, because many people are concerned about AIDS.*

Then, go on to the screening questions for HIV:

> *Are you sexually active, or have you ever injected drugs, even once?*
> *Do you have any reason to believe you are at risk for HIV?*

Follow the preceding questions, depending on whether you are talking to a man or woman, with these:

---

[1] I thank Stephen Brady, Ph.D., for suggesting many of these questions.

> *(For men): Have you had sex with a man in the past 15 years? (If yes): Can I ask what kind of sex that was? Was it oral sex or anal sex? Did you use a condom?*
> *(For women): Have you had sex with a man who sleeps with other men or who injects drugs?*
> *(For both men and women): How many sexual partners have you had over the past year?*

At this point, you've done an adequate assessment for HIV risk. You may want to follow up with some general questions about sexual functioning, which is often affected by psychiatric disorders and by the medications used to treat them.

> *Are you satisfied with your sexual functioning?*
> *Do you find that your sexual functioning changes when you get depressed (or substitute other relevant psychiatric symptom)?*

If you are interviewing someone who you suspect has been sexually abused or raped, this is a good time to ask about it.

> *Sometimes people have sex against their will. Has that ever happened to you?*
> *Have you ever been coerced into having sex?*

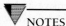

NOTES

These questions avoid the loaded terms *rape*, *molest*, and *abuse*. This is useful for patients who have been sexually coerced by a spouse or a relative and who may not want to think of their experiences in such terms.

Family Psychiatric History

The family history may be approached in one of two ways. One is the bare-bones approach, which aims to ascertain the patient's inherited risk of developing a psychiatric or medical disorder. The second approach is more extensive and is a way of beginning the social history part of the interview. I describe both approaches here and let you decide which works best for you.

BARE-BONES APPROACH

Ask the following long, high-yield question, which is adapted from a question suggested by Morrison and Munoz (2009):

> *Has any blood relative ever had nervousness, nervous breakdown, depression, mania, psychosis or schizophrenia, alcohol or drug abuse, suicide attempts, or hospitalization for nervousness?*

Because the question is so long, you have to ask it very slowly, pausing after each disorder so that the patient has time to think about it. You should also define *blood relative.*

By blood relative, I mean parents, brothers, sisters, uncles, aunts, grandparents, and cousins.

 TIP

If the patient answers with a definitive "no," you can move on. If there was a "yes," you should try to determine exactly what the diagnosis was. Unless your patient is in the mental health field and is familiar with its jargon, this may not be easy. It's helpful to ask about specific treatments the relative may have received, such as lithium, carbamazepine (Tegretol), divalproex sodium (Depakote) (clues to bipolar disorder), antipsychotics [older examples are haloperidol (Haldol) and chlorpromazine (Thorazine); newer ones are risperidone (Risperdal), olanzapine (Zyprexa), quetiapine (Seroquel), ziprasidone (Geodon), aripiprazole (Abilify), lurasidone (Latuda), and several others], electroconvulsive therapy (clue to depression, bipolar disorder, or schizophrenia, depending on when the treatment was administered), antidepressants, and antianxiety agents. Remember that medications were used differently 20 years ago. For example, in its heyday, diazepam (Valium) was given to many patients for depression, whereas now, a history of benzodiazepine treatment is a clue for the presence of an anxiety disorder.

To determine a family history of transmissible medical and neurologic problems, ask

Has any blood relative ever had a medical or neurologic illness, such as heart disease, diabetes, cancer, seizures, or senility?

How does it help diagnostically to know that a patient has a first-degree relative with a psychiatric disorder? Table 17.1 lists those psychiatric disorders for which there is significant evidence of familial transmission. The relative risk compares the risk for people with such a family history against the risk of people in the general population, who are assigned a relative risk of 1.0. For example, the relative risk of developing

TABLE 17.1. Psychiatric Disorders with Significant Evidence of Familial Transmission

DSM-5 Disorder	Lifetime Relative Risk If First-Degree Relative Has Disorder[a]	Lifetime Prevalence in General Population[b]
Bipolar I–II disorders	25	4
Schizophrenia	19	1
Bulimia nervosa	10	2[c]
Panic disorder	10	5
Alcohol abuse	7	13
Generalized anxiety disorder	6	6
Anorexia nervosa	5	1[c]
Specific phobia	3	12
Social anxiety disorder	3	12
Major depression	3	17
Obsessive-compulsive disorder	?	2[b]
Agoraphobia	3	5

[a]Relative risk figures from Reider, R. O., Kaufmann, C. A., et al. (1994). Genetics. In R. E. Hales, S. C. Yudofsky, and J. A. Talbott (Eds.), *American Psychiatric Press Textbook of Psychiatry*. Washington, DC: American Psychiatric Press. See text for explanation.

[b]Lifetime prevalence figures from Kessler, R. C., Berglund, P., Demler, O., et al. (2005). Lifetime prevalence and age-of-onset distributions of DSM-IV disorders in the national comorbidity survey replication. *Archives of General Psychiatry, 62*, 593–602.

[c]Data from Hudson, J. L., Hiripi, E., Pope, H. G., et al. (2007). The prevalence and correlates of eating disorders in the National Comorbidity Survey Replication. *Biological Psychiatry, 61*, 348–358.

bipolar disorder is 25; this means that if your patient's father is bipolar, she is 25 times more likely to develop bipolar disorder than the average person. The baseline lifetime prevalence of each disorder is also listed in the table.

Typically, family information is used in conjunction with other clinical information. For example, family history is crucial in deciding whether a patient with new-onset psychosis has schizophrenia or is in the manic phase of bipolar disorder.

THE GENOGRAM: FAMILY HISTORY AS SOCIAL HISTORY

Doing a genogram takes a while, which probably explains its lack of popularity in most clinical settings. But it doesn't take *that* long, and the time investment usually pays off in terms of richness of information. The genogram serves the additional function of introducing you to the patient's developmental history.

The technique is simple. Begin by telling your patient that you'd like to draw a family diagram to better understand her family. Draw small squares for males and circles for females. Obtain the following information about each relative:

- Age
- If dead, year, age, and cause of death (put slash mark through square or circle if dead)
- Presence of psychiatric problem, substance abuse, or major medical problem
- Status of the patient's relationship with relative (e.g., close, estranged, a perpetrator or victim of sexual or physical abuse)

Begin by diagramming the first-degree relatives, with the oldest sibling on the right (Fig. 17.1).

Once you have the skeleton of the chart, ask about each family member and embellish the chart with the information obtained. Although you will likely develop your own preferences, it is standard to write the age within the circle or square, to use slashes to represent the deceased, and to use double slashes to represent a divorce. In the example in Figure 17.2, the patient is a divorced 34-year-old man with two children who has a family psychiatric history significant for alcoholism and depression.

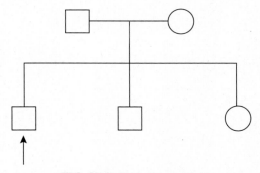

FIG. 17.1. Basic genogram.

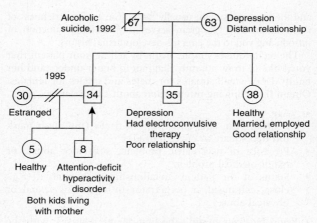

FIG. 17.2. Elaborated genogram.

Once you have completed a genogram, you have accomplished three tasks: you have obtained (a) the family psychiatric history, (b) the family medical history, and (c) the bare bones of the social and developmental history. Also, the physical layout of the genogram makes it a quick way to remind yourself of the patient's social situation, a particularly nice feature if you rarely see the patient.

18 **Obtaining the Social and Developmental History**

Essential Concepts
- Can you tell me a bit about your background, where you grew up, and how you grew up?
- Explore the following topics chronologically:
  Early family life
  School experiences, emphasizing friendships
  Work experiences
  Intimate relationships and sexual history
  Current social support network
  Goals and aspirations

Recommended time: 5 minutes

In the days when psychoanalysis was king, the social and developmental history *was* the psychiatric interview. Residents were instructed to cover everything from breast-feeding to a patient's first sexual fantasies, a process that could well take several hours. The results were written up and used to develop a psychoanalytic formulation, focusing on Freudian notions of psychosexual conflict.

In our age of psychopharmacology, interviewers sometimes reach the other extreme, asking about little more than their patient's job and marital status before moving on to the DSM-5 diagnostic questions.

What is the purpose of the social and developmental history in a brief diagnostic interview? How extensive should it be? The social history is useful in two closely related ways: (a) It allows you to get to know the patient as a *person* rather than as a *diagnosis*, and (b) you can approach the diagnosis of a personality disorder through the social history (see Chapter 31).

The essential questions take 5 minutes to ask, whereas the extended version takes 10 to 20 minutes and should be reserved for occasions on which you can take two sessions to do the evaluation.

EARLY FAMILY LIFE

Begin with the following introductory question:

> *Can you tell me a bit about your background, where you grew up, and how you grew up?*

Proceed to more specific questions, moving chronologically through the stages of life.

> *How many siblings did you have, and where were you in the birth order?*

Each family configuration has a unique impact on psychological development. Typical scenarios include the loneliness of the only child, the eldest child of a large family who was forced into the role of a parent, the ignored middle child, and the youngest child who grew up as the resented apple of his mother's eye.

> *What did your parents do for a living?*

Parental employment may have affected the patient's relationship with her parents. For example, a father who worked as a traveling salesman may not have been home much. This question also gives you a sense of socioeconomic situation: Did the patient grow up amid poverty or affluence?

> *How did you get along with your parents?*

Although there's not enough time to do this topic justice in the diagnostic interview, these questions will give you an idea of the general flavor of the home. Was it a peaceful, loving environment, or was it angry and chaotic?

> *What did they do when you disobeyed?*

This question can gently introduce the topic of physical or sexual abuse. Depending on the answer, you can follow up with a more explicit question, such as

> *Were you abused physically or sexually as you grew up?*
> *Were there any other important adults in the home?*

Often, another relative was a major factor in the patient's early life, with either a positive or a negative effect.

> *How did you get along with your siblings?*

A close relationship with siblings can often compensate for a terrible relationship with parents.

Who were you closest to, growing up?

EDUCATION AND WORK

Did you enjoy school?

This question will give you a sense of how the patient managed her first encounter with the social field outside of the family.

Did you have many friends, or did you keep to yourself?
Did you have a best friend?

The patient's lifelong pattern of relating is often apparent in the first few years of school.

What kinds of grades did you get?

Grades are a rough measure of intelligence and perseverance.

What did you do after you graduated (or dropped out)?

Did she take the straight and narrow course to college or into the job world? Or did she wander for a while, not certain what to do with her life?

Asking about Work

While I have categorized asking about work under the social and developmental history, this is often something you will ask quite early in the interview, as you are "breaking the ice." But how should you ask this question, which is a loaded one for some patients. For some patients, a straightforward "What do you do for a living" is entirely appropriate. But if you suspect that your patient may not be working, a couple of tactful inquiries are "Do you have a job or are you between jobs?" or "Are you working at the moment?" Perhaps the safest single question to ask is "How do you support yourself?" Such a question allows a patient who is on disability to reply, "I'm on disability," or allows a nonworking partner to say "My spouse brings in the money for us" (Suggestions adapted from Shea 2007).

Did you like your work?
How well did you get along with employers and colleagues?

Did the patient's pattern of relating continue unaltered as she entered the work environment?

Did she have any difficulties dealing with authority figures?

INTIMATE RELATIONSHIPS (SEXUAL HISTORY)

How does one ask about sexuality? It's always an awkward topic, and patients are usually guarded about revealing sexual information, especially when it pertains to sexual orientation. One study showed that adolescents are four times more likely to reveal a history of homosexual contact to a computer than to a person, but even the responses revealed to the computer were well below estimates of the actual prevalence of homosexuality in adolescents (Turner et al. 1996). Thus, asking about sexual history requires extra sensitivity.

Recall that in Chapter 16, I suggested some sexual history questions in the context of the medical history and the assessment of the risk for HIV. An alternative tactic is to approach these issues from within the social history. Here, the rationale for obtaining a sexual history is not so much to assess HIV risk as it is to assess the quality of the patient's intimate relationships. Is she capable of relating intimately with another? Are her intimate relationships stable or transient and chaotic, as in the case of patients with borderline personality disorder?

As with the rest of the social history, proceed chronologically:

When did you first begin dating?

Eventually, you'll decide on a way of asking about sexual orientation that is comfortable for you. The trick is to be nonjudgmental.

Were you attracted to men, women, or both?

The above question should be asked in a very matter-of-fact way, with the unspoken message that it will not faze you if the patient says that he is attracted to the same sex.

Other options are as follows:

- Precede your question with a normalizing statement, such as "Adolescents often experiment with different sexual lifestyles; was that true for you? What's your current sexual preference?"

- At the beginning of the interview, slip your question into a checklist of routine questions: "How old are you? What's your marital status? And your sexual preference?"
- Ask during the medical history when you ask about risk factors for HIV: "Do you have any risk factors for the HIV virus? Have you had homosexual sex?"

> *Are you satisfied with your sex life?*
> *Are there things about your sex life or your sexual desires that make you uncomfortable?*
> *When did you have your first important relationship?*
> *What attracted you to that person?*

Is the patient capable of establishing an intimate relationship? Can he describe other people in three-dimensional terms?

CLINICAL VIGNETTE

An attending clinician was interviewing a 40-year-old divorced man in the hospital for depression. His wife and daughter had left him 2 years earlier. He had a lifelong pattern of brief and shallow relationships. The following exchange took place as the attending clinician was exploring the relationship history:

I: Tell me about your girlfriends.
P: They were animals.
I: Pick one, and tell me about her.
P: I met a woman last year; she was a stray cat.
I: Why do you say she was a stray cat?
P: She had no connections.
I: What was it that you were attracted to?
P: Her body.
I: Okay. What kicked in about her personality later?
P: What do you mean?
I: If I met her, what would I notice about her?
P: It's tough to answer. Her attitude.
I: How was that?
P: It was good.

The patient was unable to discuss any important person in his life in more than a superficial way, which mirrored his fears of intimacy.

CURRENT ACTIVITIES AND RELATIONSHIPS

> *What attracted you to your current significant other?*
> *How has your marriage (relationship) gone?*
> *Do you have any close friends (aside from your spouse)?*
> *Are you in touch with your family?*

Does the patient have a social support system in place? Who would she call if she were in trouble?

> *What do you do during your leisure time?*

Does she enjoy sports, hobbies, reading, going to movies, and other activities, or does she only work?

> *What do you think you'll be doing 5 years from now, and what would you like to be doing?*

This question provides a window into the patient's view of her future and her dreams and aspirations.

CLINICAL VIGNETTE

An attending clinician was interviewing a 32-year-old single woman who had worked as an extremely successful attorney until a year ago, when she was fired while in the middle of a major depression. During the social history, she related that she disliked physicians in general, because her abusive father was a physician.

Toward the end of the interview, the attending clinician asked

> I: *What do you think you'll be doing in 5 years, and what would you like to be doing?*
> P: *I'll probably be dead. I'd like to be a physician.*

The attending clinician then productively explored the meaning of her seemingly paradoxical desire to become a physician.

III

INTERVIEWING FOR DIAGNOSIS: THE PSYCHIATRIC REVIEW OF SYMPTOMS

19

How to Memorize the
DSM-5 Criteria

> **Essential Concepts**
> *DSM-5* Mnemonic:
> * **D**epressed **P**atients **S**ound **A**nxious, **S**o **C**laim **P**sychiatrists
> * **D**epression and other mood disorders
> * **P**sychotic disorders
> * **S**ubstance abuse disorders
> * **A**nxiety disorders
> * **S**omatic disorders
> * **C**ognitive disorders
> * **P**ersonality disorders

Everything should be as simple as it is, but not simpler.
Albert Einstein

In this chapter, I describe an approach to memorizing the criteria for the major *DSM-5* disorders. These mnemonics are a way of sorting information into manageable chunks. Those who have researched the way expert clinicians think have found that this "chunking" process is quite common (Kaplan 2011). The father of chunking, Miller (1957), showed that humans can only process about 7 (±2) bits of information at a time, which is, presumably, why phone numbers have seven digits. You have to be able to process more than seven items to master the *DSM-5*, but mnemonics help by grouping items into information-packed chunks.

MEMORIZE THE SEVEN MAJOR DIAGNOSTIC CATEGORIES

Begin by mastering the following mnemonic for the seven major adult diagnostic categories in the *DSM-5*:

Depressed Patients Sound Anxious, So Claim Psychiatrists.
Depression and other mood disorders (major depression, bipolar disorder, dysthymia)
Psychotic disorders (schizophrenia, schizoaffective disorder, delusional disorder)

Substance abuse disorders (alcohol and drug use, psychiatric syndromes induced by drug and alcohol use)

Anxiety disorders (panic disorder, agoraphobia, generalized anxiety disorder [GAD], obsessive-compulsive disorder [OCD])

Somatic disorders (somatic symptom disorder, eating disorders)

Cognitive disorders (dementia, mental retardation, ADHD)

Personality disorders

Notice that these categories deviate somewhat from *DSM-5* dogma. For example, I call ADHD a "cognitive disorder," whereas the *DSM-5* classifies it as a "neurodevelopmental disorder." Also, I classify eating disorders under somatic disorders, whereas the *DSM-5* puts them in a separate chapter. My purpose here is not to create a new classification of psychiatric disorders but simply to rearrange them into seven categories for ease of memorization.

FOCUS ON POSITIVE CRITERIA

Now that you've memorized the major disorders, you need to memorize the diagnostic criteria. Begin by disregarding the voluminous exclusions and modifiers listed by the *DSM-5* and instead focus on the actual behaviors and affects needed to make the diagnosis.

For example, under schizophrenia in the *DSM-5* are six categories of criteria, labeled *A* through *F*. *B* is the usual proviso that the disorder must cause significant dysfunction, which is true for all the disorders, so you don't need to memorize it. *D* tells you to rule out schizoaffective and mood disorder before you diagnose schizophrenia—another obvious piece of information; don't use up valuable neurons memorizing it. *E* reminds you to rule out substance abuse or a medical condition, which you should do before making any diagnosis, and *F* deals with the arcane issue of diagnosing schizophrenia in someone who's autistic. So, only two essential criteria are left: *A* (symptoms) and *C* (duration).

This section lists mnemonics for most of the major disorders, but it does not cover how to ascertain the diagnoses, which involves the skillful use of screening questions and specific follow-up questions. These are covered in detail in Chapters 23 to 31, where the full *DSM-5* criteria are spelled out.

KEY POINT

How should you use these mnemonics? They are primarily an aid to ensure that you remember to ask about major diagnostic criteria. Do not ask the questions in the same order as the mnemonics; doing so would lead to a very stilted interview. Try to ask diagnostic questions when they seem to fit naturally into the context of the interview, using some of the techniques for making transitions already discussed in Chapters 4 and 6.

Unless stated otherwise, these mnemonics are the products of my own disordered brain.

Mood Disorders
Major Depression: SIGECAPS

Four out of these eight, with depressed mood or anhedonia, for 2 weeks signify major depression:

  Sleep disorder (either increased or decreased sleep)
  Interest deficit (anhedonia)
  Guilt (worthlessness, hopelessness, regret)
  Energy deficit
  Concentration deficit
  Appetite disorder (either decreased or increased appetite)
  Psychomotor retardation or agitation
  Suicidality

This mnemonic, devised by Dr. Carey Gross of the MGH Department of Psychiatry, refers to what might be written on a prescription sheet for a depressed, anergic patient—SIG: Energy CAPSules. Each letter refers to one of the major diagnostic criteria for a major depressive disorder. To meet the criteria for an episode of major depression, your patient must have had four of the preceding symptoms and depressed mood or anhedonia for at least 2 weeks.

Persistent Depressive Disorder (Dysthymia): ACHEWS

Two out of these six, with depressed mood, for 2 years signify persistent depressive disorder:

  Appetite disorder (either decreased or increased)
  Concentration deficit

Hopelessness
Energy deficit
Worthlessness
Sleep disorder (either increased or decreased)

The dysthymic patient is "allergic" to happiness; hence, the mnemonic refers to a dysthymic patient's (misspelled) sneezes (achoos) on exposure to happiness. To meet the criteria, the patient must have had 2 years of depressed mood with two of the six symptoms in the mnemonic.

Manic Episode: DIGFAST

Elevated mood with three of these seven, or irritable mood with four of these seven, for 1 week signify a manic episode:

Distractibility
Indiscretion (*DSM-5's* "excessive involvement in pleasurable activities…")
Grandiosity
Flight of ideas
Activity increase
Sleep deficit (decreased need for sleep)
Talkativeness (pressured speech)

I don't know who came up with this jewel, but I use it all the time. *DIGFAST* apparently refers to the speed with which a manic patient would dig a hole if put to the task. A complication in the diagnosis is that if the mood is primarily irritable, four of seven criteria must be met to qualify.

Psychotic Disorders

Schizophrenia: Delusions Herald Schizophrenic's Bad News

Requires two symptoms for 1 month, plus 5 months of prodromal or residual symptoms. At least one symptom must be one of the three highlighted core symptoms (delusions, hallucinations, speech disorganization).

Mnemonic: Delusions Herald Schizophrenic's Bad News

Delusions
Hallucinations
Speech/thought disorganization
Behavior disorganization
Negative symptoms

Substance Use Disorder

The same mnemonic, Tempted With Cognac, is used for criteria for any drug or alcohol dependence (two of the following eleven criteria are required):

- Tolerance, that is, a need for increasing amounts of alcohol to achieve intoxication
- Withdrawal syndrome
- Loss of Control of alcohol use (nine criteria follow):
  - More alcohol ingested than the patient intended
  - Unsuccessful attempts to cut down
  - Much time spent in activities related to obtaining or recovering from the effects of alcohol
  - Craving alcohol
  - Alcohol use continued despite the patient's knowledge of significant physical or psychological problems caused by its use
  - Important social, occupational, or recreational activities given up or reduced because of alcohol use
  - Failure to fulfill major role obligations at work, school, or home
  - Persistent social and interpersonal problems caused by alcohol
  - Recurrent alcohol use in situations in which it is physically hazardous

For alcohol use, the **CAGE** questionnaire is often used:

> *"Have you felt you should Cut back on your drinking?"*
> *"Has anybody Annoyed you with comments on your drinking?"*
> *"Have you felt Guilty about your drinking?"*
> *"Have you ever had an Eye-opener in the morning to get rid of a hangover?"*

Two or more affirmative answers indicate a high probability of alcohol use disorder (Ewing 1984).

Anxiety Disorders
Panic Attack (4 of 13)

With so many separate criteria to remember (13 total), trying to recall them with an acronym or phrase is not practical.

My trick instead is to break the symptoms down into three clusters: (a) the heart, (b) breathlessness, and (c) fear. To remember them, I visualize a panicking patient clutching his chest (heart cluster), hyperventilating (breathlessness cluster), and shaking with fear (fear cluster). Finally, I imagine him screaming out, "Three-five-five! Three-five-five!"—presumably as a way of distracting himself from the panic attack. The numbers refer to the number of criteria in each cluster: The heart cluster has three criteria, and the other two clusters have five each.

I admit that this all sounds hokey, but believe me, you'll never forget the criteria if you do it!

Heart Cluster: Three

I think of symptoms that often accompany a heart attack:

- Palpitations
- Chest pain
- Nausea

Breathlessness Cluster: Five

I think of symptoms associated with hyperventilation, which include dizziness, light-headedness, tingling of the extremities or lips (paresthesias), and chills or hot flashes:

- Shortness of breath
- Choking sensation
- Dizziness
- Paresthesias
- Chills or hot flashes

Fear Cluster: Five

I associate shaking and sweating with fear. To remember derealization, think of it as a way of psychologically escaping panic.

- Fear of dying
- Fear of going crazy
- Shaking
- Sweating
- Derealization or depersonalization

Aside from remembering the cluster names, remember the pattern 3-5-5 to keep from missing any of the 13 criteria. Your patient must have experienced four symptoms to meet the criteria for a full-scale panic attack.

Agoraphobia

I have no mnemonic for agoraphobia, because there are really only two criteria: a fear of being in places where escape might be difficult and efforts to avoid such places. See Chapter 25 for details.

Obsessive-Compulsive Disorder

The requirement for the diagnosis of OCD is the presence of obsessions, compulsions, or both to a degree that causes significant dysfunction. The definitions of obsessions and compulsions are easily learned and remembered (see Chapter 25), so a mnemonic is not necessary. Instead, I have chosen some of the most common symptoms seen in clinical practice; none of them is specifically required to be present by *DSM-5*.

> Washing and Straightening Make Clean Houses:
> Washing
> Straightening (ordering rituals)
> Mental rituals (e.g., magical words, numbers)
> Checking
> Hoarding (in *DSM-5*, there is now a separate "hoarding disorder")

Posttraumatic Stress Disorder

The PTSD patient Remembers Atrocious Nuclear Attacks.

> Reexperiencing the trauma via intrusive memories, flashbacks, or nightmares (**one of which is required for diagnosis**)
> Avoidance of stimuli associated with trauma
> Negative alterations in cognitions and mood (e.g., amnesia for the trauma, negative beliefs about oneself or the world, irrationally blaming oneself for the trauma, negative emotional state, restricted interests and activities, detachment, and inability to have positive emotions; **two required for diagnosis**)

Arousal increase, such as insomnia, irritability, hyper-vigilance, startle response, reckless behavior, and poor concentration (**two required for diagnosis**)

Generalized Anxiety Disorder (Three of Six)

The first part of the diagnosis of GAD is easy: The patient has worried excessively about something for 6 months. The hard part is remembering the six anxiety symptoms, three of which must be present. The following mnemonic is based on the idea that Macbeth had GAD before and after killing King Duncan:

Macbeth Frets Constantly Regarding Illicit Sins:
Muscle tension
Fatigue
Concentration problems
Restlessness, feeling on edge
Irritability
Sleep problems

If this elaborate acronym isn't to your liking, an alternative is imagining what you would experience if you were constantly worrying about something or other. You'd have **insomnia**, leading to daytime **fatigue**. Fatigue in turn would cause **irritability** and **problems concentrating**, and constant worry would cause **muscle tension** and restlessness.

Eating Disorders

Bulimia Nervosa

Bulimics Over Consume Pastries (all four of these):

Binging
Out-of-control feeling while eating
Concern with body shape
Purging

Anorexia Nervosa

Weight Fear Bothers Anorexics (all three of these):

Weight significantly low
Fear of fat
Body image distortion

Cognitive Disorders

Dementia

At least one of the following six symptoms:
Memory LAPSE

1. **Memory**
2. **L**anguage
3. **A**ttention (complex)
4. **P**erceptual-motor
5. **S**ocial cognition
6. **E**xecutive function

See Chapters 21 and 28 for further information on assessing these symptoms.

Delirium

Medical **FRAT** (all five of these):

Fluctuating course
Recent onset
Attention impairment
Thinking (cognitive) disturbance

Medical cause of cognitive impairment

Because delirium is caused by a medical illness, being part of the "medical **frat**ernity" helps to diagnose it. To merit the diagnosis, all five criteria must be present. See Chapter 28 for details.

Attention Deficit Hyperactivity Disorder

There are 18 separate, though often redundant, criteria for ADHD, making memorization impossible for anyone without a photographic memory (Table 19.1). As with panic disorder, I suggest breaking the symptoms into four broad categories, which can be remembered by the mnemonic **MOAT** (you'll need a MOAT around the classroom for the hyperactive child):

Movement excess (hyperactivity)
Organization problems (difficulty finishing tasks)
Attention problems
Talking impulsively

TABLE 19.1. *DSM-5* Criteria for ADHD

1. Six of nine disorganization/inattention symptoms or six of nine impulsivity/hyperactivity symptoms must be present.
   Disorganization/inattention symptoms:
      Organization problems
      Can't organize tasks
      Loses things needed for tasks
   Problems finishing tasks:
      Attention problems
      Poor focus
      Easily distracted
      Doesn't listen
      Forgets easily
      Makes careless mistakes
      Avoids tasks requiring concentration
      Impulsivity/hyperactivity symptoms
      Talking impulsively
      Talks too much
      Blurts out answers
      Interrupts others
      Can't play quietly
   Movement excess:
      Fidgets and squirms
      Leaves seat
      Displays restlessness
      On the go
      Can't wait for his turn
2. Some symptoms must have been present before age 12 y.
3. Symptoms occur in two or more settings, such as school (or work) and home.

Data from American Psychiatric Association. (2013). *Diagnostic and Statistical Manual of Mental Disorders* (5th ed.). Washington, DC: American Psychiatric Association.

Personality Disorders

Chapter 31 outlines a system for diagnosing personality disorders in general, including mnemonics for all ten of the personality disorders, which are not repeated here.

Interviewing for Diagnosis: The Art of Hypothesis Testing

Essential Concepts
- Use the free speech period for generating hypotheses.
- Investigate each hypothesis with screening and probing questions.
- Make graceful transitions to diagnostic questions throughout the interview.
- Use the PROS for "cleanup."

The problem is how to come up with a complete and accurate diagnosis in a very limited amount of time. Early in training, this is less of an issue, when you are encouraged to spend what you will later consider to be inordinate amounts of time interviewing your patients. But after training, you will quickly realize that there is a correlation between the number of patients that you see per day and your ability to afford a mortgage on that new home. You will be torn between the need to do things quickly and the need to do things right.

The way things are done in most busy community clinics is probably not so "right." One study compared "routine diagnoses" as found in the medical chart with a "gold standard diagnosis" generated using the SCID (Structured Clinical Interview for *Diagnostic and Statistical Manual of Mental Disorders, Revised Third Edition* [DSM-III-R]) plus chart review as well as an additional interview with a highly qualified psychiatrist or psychologist. There was only about a 50% rate of agreement between routine and gold standard diagnosis, and in one half of all cases of disagreement, feedback to the original clinicians resulted in significant changes in patient care (Ramirez Basco et al. 2000).

Does this mean that you should give the SCID to all of your patients before the interview? Thankfully not, because the techniques discussed in this section, involving screening and probing questions, mirror the SCID gold standard, adapting it to the realities of clinical practice.

One might assume that the best way to reach a diagnosis is to follow a two-step process:

1. Obtain all potentially relevant data about the patient.
2. Examine the data to determine which diagnosis fits best.

This strategy would work well if time were limitless. Because it isn't, clinicians have developed ways of determining in advance what is likely to be relevant data for a particular patient, thereby vastly increasing the efficiency of the diagnostic interview.

How do expert clinicians make diagnoses? A number of researchers have done observational studies to answer this question (Elstein et al. 1978; Kaplan 2011). They have found that experienced clinicians begin by carefully listening to the patient's initial complaint and asking open-ended questions. Based on this preliminary information, they generate a limited number of diagnostic hypotheses (the average being four) early in the interview, usually within the first 5 minutes. They then ask a number of closed-ended questions to test whether each hypothesis is true. This process is known as *pattern matching*, in which the patient's pattern of symptoms is compared with the symptom pattern required for a diagnosis.

Another way to view this approach is to think of a "closed cone" of questions (Lipkin 2002). The initial questions are open ended and exploratory; they become more closed ended to pursue a specific diagnosis to an endpoint of verification or exclusion.

In accordance with these research-based conceptions, I suggest the following four stages for rapidly establishing diagnoses during the psychiatric interview.

FREE SPEECH PERIOD

In Chapter 3, I emphasize the value of giving the patient the opening word as a way of helping to create a therapeutic alliance, but it's also valuable for beginning the process of generating hypotheses. Generating diagnoses begins the moment you first see your patient and continues throughout the interview. It's important that your mind should be especially active during the first few minutes.

Keep the mnemonic "**D**epressed **P**atients **S**ound **A**nxious, **S**o **C**laim **P**sychiatrists" in mind as you listen to your patient. Does she appear depressed or manic? Is she speaking coherently, and is her reality testing good? Does she seem anxious? Does she seem sharp or cognitively impaired? Is she beginning the interview complaining of numerous somatic symptoms? Does she have alcohol on her breath? Does she seem inappropriately angry or entitled? You will quickly be able to generate a mental list of likely diagnoses, which you should follow up on later in the interview with appropriate screening and probing questions.

SCREENING AND PROBING QUESTIONS

Once you've generated your short list of likely diagnoses, go on to test your hypotheses. Begin by asking a screening question that gets at the core feature of the disorder. Each disorder-specific chapter in Section III suggests one or more screening questions. For instance, a screening question for bipolar disorder (see Chapter 24) is

> *Have you ever had a period of a week or so when you felt so happy and energetic that your friends said that you were talking too fast or that you were behaving differently and strangely?*

If the patient answers "yes," go right into the mnemonic for manic episodes (DIGFAST) and ask primarily closed-ended questions about each criterion. If the patient answers "no" and you are certain that he understood the question, you should conclude that bipolar disorder is unlikely and move onto another part of the interview.

Interviewing for diagnosis is an active, probing process in which you will often do as much talking as your patient. Is such an active style really more effective in eliciting diagnostic information than a quieter, listening style? Common sense dictates that it is, and the Maudsley Hospital researchers concluded that it is as well. In one of their papers examining techniques for eliciting factual information (Cox et al. 1981b), they found that a focused and directive style, in which interviewers used many probing questions and often requested detailed information, led to better data than did a more passive style. The best data were obtained when interviewers used at least nine probing questions per symptom. Data were judged to be "better" when, in addition to the mere mention of a symptom, such as depression, interviewers could obtain information about the frequency, duration, severity, context, and qualities of the symptom, all of which are extremely important for diagnostic decision making.

The concern remains that a directive style may elicit great factual data at the expense of shutting the patient down emotionally with too much questioning and not enough listening. Cox et al. (1981a) examined this issue and found that more directive interviewers actually elicited slightly more feelings than did interviewers with a less directive style.

TRANSITION GRACEFULLY TO DIAGNOSTIC QUESTIONS

 KEY POINT

Don't try to turn the diagnostic interview into a long checklist of diagnostic questions. This gives the interview a mechanical feeling and will diminish patient rapport. Instead, ask diagnostic questions at relevant points in the interview, using the transition skills you learned in Chapter 6. Much of Section III gives you tips for accomplishing such transitions; here are a few examples as a preview.

Illustrative Transitions to Diagnostic Areas

* Depression
  With things so bad in your marriage, I wonder how it's been affecting your mood.
* OCD
  You said you're often late. Are there rituals you do at home that make you late, like checking or cleaning things?
* Substance abuse
  Given all the stress you've been under, do you have a drink now and then to deal with it?
* Suicidality
  With things going so poorly in your life, I wonder if you've been debating whether it's worth it to go on?

- Borderline personality disorder
  Earlier you mentioned that your husband left you years ago; how do you normally deal with rejection?
- Psychosis
  You've been through so much stress lately—does it ever cause your mind to play tricks on you, so that you hear voices or have strange ideas?

PSYCHIATRIC REVIEW OF SYMPTOMS

 TIP

It's not uncommon to forget to ask important questions during an interview, even if you use all the mnemonics in Chapter 19. The PROS is a helpful way to prevent this from happening. At some point toward the end of the interview, mentally review the *DSM-5* mnemonic (**D**epressed **P**atients **S**ound **A**nxious, **S**o **C**laim **P**sychiatrists) and ask screening questions for any disorder that you haven't yet explored. This step resembles the survey approach that I decried earlier, but it's usually quite brief, because by this time you already will have covered the priority topics.

The PROS is usually best begun with an introduced transitional statement, such as

Now, I'd like to switch gears a little and ask you about a bunch of different psychological symptoms some people have.

Mental Status Examination

> **Essential Concepts**
> Mnemonic for Elements of the Mental Status Examination:
>
> **A**ll **B**orderline **S**ubjects **A**re **T**ough, **T**roubled **C**haracters
> **ABSATTC**
> - **A**ppearance
> - **B**ehavior
> - **S**peech
> - **A**ffect
> - **T**hought process
> - **T**hought content
> - **C**ognitive examination

Nothing in the psychiatric assessment is as misunderstood as the mental status examination (MSE). Two misconceptions are ubiquitous. The first is that the MSE takes place at the particular point in the interview when you test orientation and recall. In fact, the MSE occurs throughout the entire interview, during which you are constantly evaluating affect, concentration, memory, and insight. The second myth is that the MSE is identical to the Folstein Mini-Mental State Examination (MMSE). In fact, the Folstein MMSE is a specific screen for dementia. Increasingly, its use in the routine psychiatric interview is being questioned, but we'll talk more about that later.

The MSE is your evaluation of your patient's current state of cognitive and emotional functioning. Although most of the initial interview is specifically focused on your patient's past, doing an excellent MSE requires that you attend at the same time to his present. Here, your "third ear" comes into play. How is your patient presenting himself? What is his TP like? How is he emoting? It will take you years to hone your powers of observation, and this is certainly the most interesting part of the diagnostic interview.

An MSE accomplishes two purposes. First, it helps make a diagnosis, especially in those cases in which historical data are unreliable or equivocal. A patient could send you an e-mail listing all of his depressive symptoms, but it requires direct observation—an MSE—to assess the degree of his anguish and his need for treatment. Second, the MSE allows you to create a vivid patient description for your records. Using this, you can more easily track your patient's progress from visit to visit, and you can give clinicians to whom you refer a more accurate sense of his condition.

ELEMENTS OF THE MENTAL STATUS EXAMINATION

The MSE has roughly seven components. This mnemonic will help you to remember them:

All Borderline Subjects Are Tough, Troubled Characters:

Appearance
Behavior
Speech
Affect
Thought process
Thought content
Cognitive examination

Appearance

How does your patient's appearance help you in your evaluation? At the extremes, a specific diagnosis might immediately suggest itself. For example, a disheveled man wearing bizarrely mismatched layers of clothes is schizophrenic until proven otherwise. Likewise, a flamboyant and seductively dressed woman with bright makeup who bounces into your office with energy to spare strongly suggests mania.

In usual clinical practice, however, these pathognomonic presentations are rare, and appearance provides more subtle, but no less useful, information. Qualities to note include

- Self-esteem: Does the patient care about his appearance? Compare the following two patient descriptions:

  The patient was a mildly overweight man with unruly black curly hair, dressed in ill-fitting baggy jeans and a T-shirt so tight that his stomach was visibly bulging above his belt.

  The patient was a slim man who appeared younger than his 47 years, with fashionably cut short brown hair, an ironed button-down shirt, new jeans, and polished penny loafers.

Both patients were diagnosed with depression, but they presented very differently and required different treatment plans.

- Personal statement: Does the appearance say something specific about your patient's interests, activities, or attitudes?

  The patient came into the office dressed in a pressed electrician's uniform, with his name stitched over his breast pocket.

  She wore a T-shirt with the slogan, "Every day I'm forced to add one more name to the list of people who piss me off."

- Memorable aspects: Describe whatever particularly strikes you about your patient. For example, if he is particularly attractive, note it, since degree of attractiveness is usually relevant to self-image. However, I have yet to see any report describe a patient as "unattractive," and I wouldn't recommend it, because it implies that you disliked him. Instead, describe the unattractive aspects.

  This was a man of normal build who had a round, acne-covered face and was essentially bald, with the exception of small amounts of oily black hair on either side.

  Sometimes, a particular feature jumps out at you:

  She had short curly brown hair, and her left eye was congenitally deviated toward the left, giving her a somewhat unsettling appearance.

TIP

The more vivid the notation, the better. I find it helpful to actually jot down a few descriptors at the beginning of the interview, during the free speech period.

Comment on height and build; hair color, style, and quality, including facial hair, if any; facial features, including eyes; clothes; movements; and any other prominent features of appearance, like tattoos or scars.

Table 21.1 (included in Appendix A as a pocket card) may appear to restate the obvious, but it's useful to me when I lack the right descriptive words.

TABLE 21.1. Appearance Terms

Aspect of Appearance	Descriptors
Hair	Bald, thinning, close cropped, short, long, shoulder length, crew cut, straight, curly, wavy, frizzy, braided, pony tail, pig tails, afro, relaxed, dreadlocks, unevenly cut, stiff, greasy, dry, matted
Facial hair	Clean shaven, neatly trimmed beard, long and scraggly beard, goatee, unshaven
Face	Attractive, nice looking, pleasant, plain, pale, drawn, ruddy, flushed, bony, thin, broad, moon shaped, red nosed, thickly made up
Eyes	(Gaze) Good or poor eye contact, shifty, averted gaze, staring, fixated, dilated, downcast, forceful, intense, aggressive, piercing
Body	Thin, cachectic, lean, frail, underweight, normal build, muscular, husky, stocky, overweight, moderately obese, obese, morbidly obese, short, medium height, tall, tattooed arms
Movements	No abnormal movements, fidgety, bobbing knee, facial tic or twitch, lip smacking, lip puckering, tremulous, jittery, restless, wringing hands, motionless, rigid, limp, stiff, slumped
Clothes	Casually dressed, neat, appropriate, professional, immaculate, fashionable, sloppy, ill fitting, outdated, flamboyant, sexually provocative, soiled, dirty, tight, loose, slogans on clothes

Behavior and Attitude

How did your patient behave toward you when you first met her? Was she friendly and cooperative, or did she seem indifferent and apathetic? Did she sit right down and face you, or was she agitated, pacing around the room and talking rapidly without really attending to your questions? The context of the interview may also be important to making sense of the behavior. Was it a scheduled evaluation interview or did it take place in an emergency room?

Descriptors of attitude are similar to descriptors of affect (Table 21.2), but the emphasis is on words that describe a relationship toward someone. Often, a sentence of description is important. Here are some examples:

> *He presented himself as someone who was very anxious to tell his story and to gain relief from his symptoms. He had an attitude of submissive respect, saying things like, "Do you think you can help me, doctor? What do you think I have?"*
> *She presented as indifferent and apathetic. Her general attitude was that this was just the latest in a long string of unhelpful interviews.*

Often, your patient's attitude toward you will change over the course of the interview.

TABLE 21.2. Affect Terms

Affect	Terms
Normal	Appropriate, calm, pleasant, relaxed, normal, friendly, comfortable, unremarkable
Happy	Cheerful, bright, peppy, content, self-satisfied, silly, giggly, grandiose, euphoric, elated, exalted
Sad	Sad, gloomy, sullen, depressed, pessimistic, morose, hopeless, discouraged
Anxious	Anxious, worried, tense, nervous, apprehensive, frightened, terrified, bewildered, paranoid
Angry	Angry, irritable, disdainful, bitter, arrogant, defensive, sarcastic, annoyed, furious, enraged, hostile
Indifferent	Indifferent, shallow, superficial, cool, distant, apathetic, aloof, dull, vacant, affectless, uninterested, cynical

He was initially reluctant to answer questions and seemed irritable. Over the course of the interview, he became more self-revealing and tearful.

Speech

Description of speech has great overlap with description of TP, because we can only know our patients' thoughts through speech. Qualities of speech to consider include

* Rate: Does he speak rapidly or slowly? Rapid or "pressured" speech is usually a buzzword for manic speech, but you need to be careful not to overpathologize. Rapid speech can signal anxiety or even be the normal speech pattern. We all know people who speak very rapidly but are not manic.
* Volume: Patients who speak loudly may be manic, irritable, or anxious. Very low volume may signal depression or shyness. Again, loud or quiet speech may also be a nonpathologic variant of normal.
* Latency of response: Normally, when you are asked a question, you'll think for a fraction of a second before responding. This is the normal latency of response. Manic patients may respond so quickly that they seem to jump onto the last few words of your questions. Depressed or psychotic patients may show an increased latency of response, waiting several seconds before answering simple questions.
* General quality: Does your patient speak thoughtfully and in an articulate manner, or does she ramble in a vague and disconnected way, making her hard to follow? The terms in Table 21.3 are discussed in more detail in Chapter 27, in the section on disorders of TP.

Affect and Mood

Traditional teaching distinguishes mood from affect, with *mood* defined as a patient's subjective report of how he feels, and *affect* defined as your own impression of his emotional

TABLE 21.3. Speech Terms

Normal
Thoughtful
Articulate
Intelligent
Rapid
Staccato
Pressured
Rambling
Continuous
Loud
Soft
Barely audible
Slow
Halting

state. Although many clinicians do not make this distinction in clinical work, you should become familiar with it, because it is widely used.

Like observation of appearance and behavior, accurate observation of affect is a skill that takes years to master. Although the overall emotional flavor is usually obvious, the gradations and subtleties are not, and assessing degree of affect can be vitally important for such things as determining imminence of SI or predicting the likelihood of aggressive acting out.

Often, you won't have to explicitly ask your patient how he's been feeling, because he'll report it spontaneously. However, what do you do when your patient is vague about his emotions or is reluctant to reveal himself?

The obvious (and easiest) approach is to come right out and ask.

> How do you feel right now? How has your mood been over the past few days?

If the patient answers with a vague term, follow up with questions aimed at giving a more refined name to the affect, a name on which you both can agree but which you have not "fed" the patient.

CLINICAL VIGNETTE

> *Interviewer: How have you been feeling over the past few days?*
> *Patient: Not so great.*
> *Interviewer: Hmmm. Not so great. Can you give that feeling a name?*
> *Patient: Just… really lousy.*
> *Interviewer: I mean an emotion word, like sad, nervous, angry, and so on.*
> *Patient: Sad, I guess.*

One particularly difficult situation is when your patient says he feels "up and down" or that he has "mood swings." Suddenly you are faced with a huge diagnostic differential. Does the patient have bipolar disorder? Cyclothymia? Does he have depression with mood reactivity? Does he have a personality disorder? An anxiety disorder? A substance use disorder? All of these are compatible with an up-and-down mood.

Your questioning strategy should be based on trying to locate an enduring, persistent mood beneath the variations. Or, if there is true mood instability, you should determine whether the lows meet criteria for major depression and the highs satisfy criteria for mania. I'll have more to say about these issues in Chapters 23 and 24, but here's an example of a strategy that usually works well:

CLINICAL VIGNETTE

> *Interviewer: How have you been feeling over the past few days?*
> *Patient: (Shaking head, looking at interviewer intensely.) Totally up and down.*
> *Interviewer: Tell me about the downs first. When you say "down," do you mean sad or depressed, or something else?*
> *Patient: Really depressed.*
> *Interviewer: Do you feel depressed nearly every day?*
> *Patient: Sometimes I get really happy.*

Interviewer: I want to talk about the happy times, too, in a second. To focus on the down times, do you have depressed periods nearly every day?
Patient: Yes.
Interviewer: Is your concentration affected during those depressed periods?

[The interviewer goes through the neurovegetative symptoms (NVSs) of depression and determines that the patient meets criteria for a major depressive episode.]

Interviewer: Now, tell me more about the really happy times you've been having. What do you mean by "ups"?
Patient: Feeling great, feeling on top of the world.
Interviewer: Okay. Do you really feel great nearly every day?
Patient: No, not every day, but sometimes I do.
Interviewer: Over the past 2 weeks, how many days would you say you felt really great?
Patient: Oh, a couple. My parents gave me a car for graduation. I was so happy.
Interviewer: How long did that happy mood last?
Patient: Couple of days.
Interviewer: Then how did you feel?
Patient: Down, as usual.

The eventual diagnosis was major depression, because the patient's pervasive mood had been depression, with a number of the required NVSs. The "ups" turned out to be brief reprieves from the persistent depressed mood.

Table 21.2 (included as a pocket card in Appendix A) is a useful reference while you're writing up the MSE. Use it to enrich your emotional vocabulary, so that you don't get in the habit of using a single word to describe all patients with a particular kind of affect.

Qualities of Affect

Four qualities of affect are commonly taught, but, as with the distinction between mood and affect, the usefulness of these distinctions is controversial. My opinion is that there is too much hairsplitting in academic psychiatry and that clinical work would be simpler and just as effective without worrying about the following distinctions. Nonetheless, many would disagree, and you should at least become familiar with the terms, whether or not you use them.

1. *Stability of affect:* This refers to a continuum from *stable* affect (generally defined as normal) to *labile* affect (generally abnormal). Marked lability of affect (e.g., when a patient alternates between giggling and uncontrollable sobbing) is usually a marker of either mania or acute psychosis, but it may also be seen in dementia and other neuropsychiatric syndromes.

2. *Appropriateness:* A patient who laughs uncontrollably while talking about her mother's death is exhibiting inappropriate affect, and this is useful to record. Inappropriate affect is often seen in psychosis or mania. Don't over-pathologize, however; many intact people smile a bit when talking about sad things. This may reflect a defense mechanism such as denial, rather than psychosis.

3. *Range of affect:* Mentally healthy humans exhibit a full range of affect. At some moments they feel happy, at other moments annoyed, and at others sad. Depressed patients are said to exhibit *constricted* affect, and patients with schizophrenia are often said to exhibit *flat* affect. The problem, of course, is that many healthy people exhibit a narrow range of affect. This may be especially true during a psychiatric interview, because patients may not feel emotionally safe exposing themselves to a stranger. Thus, the diagnostic specificity of a limited range of affect is suspect and should not be overinterpreted.

4. *Intensity of affect:* Intensity is often hard to distinguish from range of affect, and like range, the diagnostic specificity is unknown. The usual jargon describes three grades: intense, flat, and blunted. *Flat* and *blunted* are usually reserved for descriptions of severely depressed patients or patients with negative symptoms of schizophrenia. *Intense* is often used for manic or histrionic patients, but remember that many completely healthy people come across as passionate or intense.

Thought Process

TP refers to the flow of thought (coherent vs. incoherent) and is covered in detail in Chapter 27.

Thought Content

Thought content (TC) refers to unusual or dangerous ideas and includes SI and homicidal ideation (HI) (see Chapter 22); psychotic ideation, such as delusions and hallucinations (see Chapter 27); and any significant themes that came up during the interview and relate to the psychiatric diagnosis.

Cognitive Examination

What are the essential components of the screening cognitive examination? There is no general agreement on this issue, and many clinicians argue that much of what is commonly taught as essential to the cognitive examination is of questionable use (Rapp 1979). For example, most training programs continue to teach the serial sevens subtraction test (SSST) of attention, even though studies have demonstrated that it has little validity in separating demented patients from healthy patients. (See the section on Attention and Concentration for a more complete discussion.) Many of the other commonly taught elements of the cognitive examination are equally suspect, including the digit span test, abstractions, similarities, proverbs, and judgment questions (Keller and Manschreck 1989).

I focus here on what is truly useful in helping you to differentiate between normal and impaired cognition. You should be aware, however, that this is a screening approach only. Specialized tests of cognitive abilities, usually conducted by a neuropsychologist, should be done if your screening indicates a potential problem.

▼ **Caveat:** Studies have shown that low educational attainment correlates with poor performance on cognitive testing in the absence of dementia or other organic impairments (Manly et al. 1999; Murden et al. 1991). Most studies have defined *poorly educated* as 8 or fewer years of education—that is, no high school. The implication for clinicians is that you should ask about educational level before testing and be cautious about overinterpreting cognitive abnormalities in poorly educated patients.

The elements of cognition that you should assess include

- Level of awareness or wakefulness
- Attention and concentration

- Memory
- Judgment
- Insight

Perception is important too, of course, but its assessment is discussed in Chapter 27.

Level of Awareness or Wakefulness

KEY POINT

The continuum of wakefulness ranges from comatose to fully alert. Determining the level of wakefulness is important for two reasons. First, it will clue you in to certain diagnoses, such as benzodiazepine or alcohol abuse in the drowsy patient or mania or stimulant abuse in the hyperalert patient. Second, it will give you guidance in how to proceed with the rest of the cognitive examination. For example, a full cognitive examination is not valid in a patient who is nodding off throughout the interview.

The assessment of wakefulness is easy enough. Your first 10 seconds of contact with a patient will tell you whether he is alert enough to greet you appropriately and tell you his name. If he seems sleepy, you have at your disposal an entire lexicon for describing degrees of sleepiness: sleepy, drowsy, lethargic, somnolent, stuporous, obtunded, and comatose. Because there are no generally agreed-on definitions of most of these terms, it's best to describe the degree of sleepiness in plain English. Thus, instead of "stuporous," say:

> *The patient was sleepy and could only be awakened by my calling his name loudly and shaking his shoulder.*

Instead of "drowsy," say:

> *The patient yawned frequently during the interview but attended well to all questions.*
> *The patient nodded off frequently and had difficulty resuming his train of thought.*

These descriptions help the reader of your assessment to draw conclusions regarding the reliability of the rest of the MSE.

Attention and Concentration

You want to assess whether your patient can sustain attention over a period of time. The continuum of attention runs from attentive and focused at one end to confused and distractible at the other.

Most training programs teach two tests for assessing attention: the digit span test and the SSST. In the digit span test, the patient is given five to seven numbers and asked to repeat them forward and backward; in the SSST, the patient is asked to subtract seven from 100 and to continue counting back by sevens until told to stop. Both of these tasks intuitively seem like reasonable tests of attention; however, research studies have not endorsed them.

In one study (Smith 1967), the SSST was given to 132 normal adults aged 18 to 63, all of whom were fully employed and the majority of whom had at least 16 years of education. The professions represented included psychiatry, psychology, neurology, and pediatrics. Only 42% of these subjects had errorless performance on the SSST. Fully, 31 of the subjects made between 3 and 12 errors, and 14 either gave stereotyped responses (supposedly consistent with frontal lobe disease) or totally abandoned the task. In another study (Milstein et al. 1972), 325 hospitalized psychiatric patients were given the SSST. No difference in performance between patients and 50 healthy control subjects appeared, and there was no association between poor performance on the test and the presence of organic cognitive impairments. With regard to the digit span test, Crook et al. (1980) found no difference in seven-digit recall among 60 elderly patients who had memory impairment and 44 elderly people who were healthy.

On the other hand, the months backward test (MBT), in which you ask the patient to recite all 12 months in reverse, appears to be fairly sensitive. The vast majority of cognitively normal adults can complete the test accurately in about 20 seconds, and any errors of omission are strongly suggestive of cognitive impairment (Meagher et al. 2015). Simply ask your patient to recite the months backward, beginning with December.

TIP

The best way to assess attention and concentration is simply to talk to your patient and observe how she thinks. Is she able to concentrate on your questions? Can she maintain a train of thought as she answers you? If the answer to these questions is "yes," your patient's attention is intact.

Memory

You should assess both short-term memory (memory of things learned a few minutes to a few days ago) and long-term memory (memory of things learned longer than a few days ago). Studies have documented that the most clinically valid tests of these are (a) orientation, (b) three-object recall, (c) recall of remote personal events, and (d) recall of general cultural information (Keller and Manschreck 1989).

Orientation

Orientation to person, place, and time is often thought to be a specific test of delirium or confusion, but it is actually a test of memory. One's name, one's location, and the date are all pieces of information that must be learned and retained. Whereas one's name is invariant and therefore is encoded in long-term memory, both the date and the place change often, offering ideal ways to test whether people are capable of retaining new information.

Because asking people where they are and what the date is can feel awkward, here are some ways to transition into these questions smoothly. You can introduce all your memory questions with a statement such as

> I'd like to change gears here and ask you a few questions to test your memory.

Often, you can make a smooth transition from some information you just obtained:

> (The patient just told you her father had Alzheimer's disease.) Speaking of that, how has your memory been? I'd like to ask you some questions to test your memory.

(The patient said his concentration has been poor while he's been depressed.) Speaking of concentration, I'd like to ask a few questions to test how your memory and concentration are doing now.

Once you've introduced the need to assess memory, you can go into your orientation questions with a question such as

Do you keep track of time pretty well?

Regardless of the response, you can follow up with

For example, would you be able to tell me today's date?

 TIP

If your patient is taking a while and struggling to remember, a time-saving tip is to ask about specific components, going from easiest to hardest.

What year is it? What month? What day of the week? And what's the date?

▼ **Caveat:** Don't overinterpret an inaccurate date. Many cognitively intact people don't keep close track of the date. To prove this to yourself, ask yourself what the date is today. If you're off by a day, you're normal. Thus, in recording your MSE, rather than writing "patient was not oriented to date," record instead what the patient said. Assuming, for example, that the true date is Monday, November 30, 2015, there is a world of difference between the patient who says "Monday, November 29, 2015," and the patient who answers, "sometime in '98."

Three-Object Recall

Recall of three objects after at least 2 minutes has been shown to be a useful test in diagnosing cognitive impairments (Hinton and Withers 1971). Say to your patient:

Repeat the following three words: ball, chair, purple.

Make sure your patient can repeat them correctly before moving on. You must be satisfied that your patient has correctly registered all three of the words, because otherwise your test of memory will not be valid. Some elderly patients may have difficulty repeating the words because of a hearing problem. (One of my hard-of-hearing patients repeated the words as "pall, share, gurgle.") In such cases, repeat the words more loudly until they have registered. You may encounter a similar problem if English is not your patient's first language. Of course, if your patient is extremely demented or confused, she will not be able to repeat the words for that reason. However, patients with such severe cognitive impairment will have already been diagnosed because of difficulties in answering basic informational questions early in the interview.

Once you are satisfied that your patient has registered all three words, say:

> *Now I want you to remember those three words, because I'm going to ask you to repeat them in a couple of minutes.*

In the meantime, ask your patient general knowledge questions (see below) about general cultural and personal information. Then ask him to repeat the three words.

If your patient has trouble, use the following hints:

> *One of them is something you can play with.*
> *One is a piece of furniture.*
> *One is a color.*

Cognitively, normal people usually remember all three words, and if they forget one, they will remember it after your hint. Performance any worse than that indicates a possible problem in short-term memory.

General Cultural Knowledge

Certain items of cultural and historical information have been so widely taught that you can assume any American with at least a high school education has learned them. Inability to recall at least half of these items is presumptive evidence of long-term memory impairment.

TIP

The traditional task is to name the last five presidents, although there's no evidence that there is anything magical about the number five. In practice, cognitively intact patients may have problems remembering that George Bush came before Clinton and that Reagan came before Bush. Therefore, I recommend asking about the last *three* presidents.

- Last three presidents: Begin with

  Who is the current president?

- Then

  Who was president before Obama?
  Who was before George W. Bush?

- Other famous figures: I ask about people who are so enduringly famous that the average person can't get through a typical month without hearing a reference to them.

  Who was_____? What was he/she famous for?

- Here are a few of these famous people, along with what a cognitively intact person should be able to tell you about them:

  George Washington, first president
  Abraham Lincoln, freed the slaves
  Martin Luther King, Jr., civil rights leader
  Princess Diana, British princess killed in car accident
  William Shakespeare, writer
  Christopher Columbus, discovered America

- Famous dates: In asking these questions, you should not expect a precisely correct response, but rather a response that names a year in the ballpark.

  When did World War II happen? (Any time in the 1930s or 1940s is adequate.)
  When was John F. Kennedy assassinated? (Sometime in the 1960s.)

- Lists of information: A highly sensitive approach to screening for dementia is the *set test*, first described in 1973 (Isaacs and Kennie 1973). The procedure is to ask your patient to name as many items (up to ten) as he can recall in each of four categories: colors, animals, fruits, and towns. Out of a maximum of 40, a score of 25 or above excluded the diagnosis of dementia in the original study.

Personal Knowledge

Personal knowledge includes aspects of current life as well as memory of remote personal events. Cognitively intact patients should be able to tell you

- Current address and phone number
- Names and ages of spouse, siblings, and children
- Spouse's birthday, wedding anniversary, and date and place of marriage (if married)
- Parents' names and birthdays (primarily for younger patients who are not married)

TIP

How do you know if the patient's answer is accurate? Address, phone number, and spouse's name are often on the chart's registration sheet. You can check the other information by calling a family member. Generally, however, patients do not blatantly confabulate, alcoholic dementia being the major exception to this, and you can often get a sense of cognitive status without resorting to time-consuming phone calls.

Intelligence

As with concentration, you can get a general idea of level of intelligence via the rest of the interview. Think of intelligence as the ability to manipulate information. High levels of educational and job attainment usually correlate with high intelligence.

TIP

For a quick and dirty measure of intelligence quotient (IQ), you can give the easy-to-remember Wilson Rapid Approximate Intelligence Test (Wilson 1967) (Table 21.4). Start with 2 × 48 as a screening test. If the patient can calculate this, she's very unlikely to be in the borderline or retarded range, and you can end the testing. Patients who can't calculate 2 × 24 are likely to meet IQ criteria for mental retardation and should definitely be referred for formal neuropsychological testing. The usual caveat regarding educational level applies: You should only give this test to patients who have completed high school.

Insight

KEY POINT

Although the term *insight* has many layers of meaning, for the purposes of the evaluation interview, you are most interested in whether your patient knows that he has an illness and has some realistic conception of its causes and possible treatments.

Sometimes, a patient's lack of insight is blatant. Such is the case with many patients with mania and schizophrenia, who may be absolutely convinced of the veracity of their

TABLE 21.4. Wilson Rapid Approximate Intelligence Test

Intelligence	Best Effort	IQ (Rough Estimate)
Retarded	2 × 6	<70
Borderline	2 × 24	70–80
Dull normal	2 × 48	80–90
Average	2 × 384	90–110
Bright normal	2 × 1,536	110–120
Superior	2 × 3,072	120–130

delusions. Documenting poor insight in such cases is easy, but in many cases, you have to probe for degree of insight by asking, often toward the end of the interview:

> So, why do you think you've been having these problems?
> What do you think needs to happen for your life to improve?

Insightful patients will be able to identify some psychosocial stressors related to their disorder (either as cause or effect). Patients with poor insight might respond with phrases such as:

> I don't know. You're the doctor.
> People need to stop hassling me. (A paranoid patient.)

Whereas complete lack of insight is often seen in psychotic disorders or dementia, poor insight might point you at a diagnosis of a character disorder or low intelligence.

Judgment

The standard question for testing judgment is by now widely recognized as unhelpful in assessing the sort of judgment in which clinicians are interested:

> If you found a stamped and addressed envelope laying on the sidewalk, what would you do?

Instead, you should assess judgment based on the material gathered throughout the interview. Did your patient decide to seek help when she felt depressed? Did she apply for unemployment benefits when she lost her job? These show good judgment. Did she decide that the best treatment for her depression was to go on a cocaine binge? This shows poor judgment.

Often, students lump tests of abstraction with tests of judgment. These include the interpretation of proverbs and the recognition of similarities. These tests show very low interrater reliability (Andreasen et al. 1974), they show no demonstrated usefulness in the diagnosis of organic problems, and good performance is highly correlated with intelligence (Keller and Manschreck 1989), which is generally not what the tests are supposed to be testing.

SHOULD YOU USE THE FOLSTEIN MINI-MENTAL STATE EXAMINATION?

The Folstein MMSE (Folstein et al. 1975) contains 11 categories of scored questions. The maximum possible score is 30, and scores below 30 may indicate cognitive impairment, with the precise cutoff point varying by age and education. The sensitivity of the test is high—you're unlikely to miss cases of dementia—but the specificity is low, meaning that many patients who are cognitively healthy will be misclassified as demented. This happened in 17% of patients in one study (Anthony et al. 1982).

Whether the MMSE should be used in all psychiatric evaluations is a matter of great controversy. Opponents argue that the test's positive predictive value is unacceptably low and that it is less sensitive and specific than clinical judgment that is based on the results of the entire interview (Harwood et al. 1997; Tangalos et al. 1996). Proponents argue that its high sensitivity makes it essential and that a numerical measure of cognitive functioning is a great help in tracking the course of dementia. But even the usefulness of the MMSE for tracking cognitive decline has come into question. Researchers examined a large registry of patients with Alzheimer's disease and followed MMSE scores over several years. Although they found that there was a 3.4-point average annual decline, the measurement error of the test was almost as large (2.8), and even after 4 years of follow-up, 15.8% of patients had no clinically meaningful decline in the MMSE score.

The MMSE is most useful for clinicians with little training in the psychiatric interview who need a standardized format for asking a series of questions. It is less useful for mental health clinicians, because we can skillfully ascertain cognitive functioning from the interview as a whole and can target particular questions to assess specific areas of possible impairment. In addition, the MMSE includes one test that has been found to be invalid for evaluating cognitive impairment (SSST) and does *not* include other questions that are very important in assessing for dementia, such as questions about personal and general knowledge.

Notwithstanding the many limitations of the MMSE, it is used so widely in a variety of clinical settings that you should become familiar with it.

MINI-COG

A more recent streamlined dementia screen, called the Mini-Cog, has been validated and is easy and quick to administer. This combines two tests: the three-item recall (of MMSE fame) and the clock-drawing task (CDT). Studies comparing the Mini-Cog with the MMSE have shown no real differences in sensitivity or specificity, and the Mini-Cog is much faster to administer and avoids most of the cultural and language problems associated with the MMSE (Tsoi et al. 2015).

The Mini-Cog is administered in two steps. First, you ask your patient if you can test his memory by asking him to repeat and memorize three simple words (the specific words are up to you). Then you give him a paper and pen and ask him to draw a clock, with the hands pointing to "11:10" (or pick another time in which there is a hand on each side of the clock). Once the clock is drawn, ask him to repeat your three words.

How do you interpret your patient's performance? Use the results of the three-item recall as a screen. Patients who recall all three words are not demented, those who can remember none of them are demented, whereas those who remember one or two might be demented. For patients in the middle, their performance on the CDT provides crucial information that may or may not convince you to seek neuropsychological testing.

Assessing Suicidal and Homicidal Ideation

> **Essential Concepts**
>
> Suicidal Ideation
> - Learn the **SAD PERSONS** risk factors for suicide.
> - Use the **CASE** approach for assessing suicide risk.
> - Assess passive suicidality.
> - Assess active suicidality.
> - Assess imminent plan.
>
> Homicidal Ideation
> - Learn the risk factors for homicide.
> - Ask about HI.
> - Know your Tarasoff duties.

We cannot tear out a single page from our life, but we can throw the whole book into the fire.

George Sand

RISK FACTORS FOR SUICIDE

The reason an assessment of suicidality is necessary in every diagnostic interview is obvious enough: We hope to prevent suicide. However, the mental health field has not yet devised tools that allow prediction of suicidal behavior in a particular patient. On the other hand, researchers have discovered a number of factors that increase the statistical risk for suicide. It is important to be aware of these risk factors as you interview any potentially suicidal patient.

In evaluating suicidality during the initial interview, you have two goals. The first and most important is to assess whether an immediate risk of a suicide attempt exists. Your second goal is to determine current or past suicidality to help you formulate an accurate *DSM-5* diagnosis. You can achieve both of these goals with the same line of questioning.

Before reviewing the types of questions to ask, you should be familiar with the risk factors for suicide. An excellent mnemonic for the major risk factors is "**SAD PERSONS**," devised by Patterson et al. (1983).

Mnemonic: SAD PERSONS (risk factors for suicide):

Sex: Women are more likely to attempt suicide; men are more likely to succeed.

Age: Age falls into a bimodal distribution, with teenagers and the elderly at highest risk.

Depression: Fifteen percent of depressive patients die by suicide.

Previous attempt: Ten percent of those who have previously attempted suicide die by suicide.

Ethanol abuse: Fifteen percent of alcoholics commit suicide.

Rational thinking loss: Psychosis is a risk factor, and 10% of patients with chronic schizophrenia die by suicide.

Social supports are lacking.

Organized plan: A well-formulated suicide plan is a red flag.

No spouse: Being divorced, separated, or widowed is a risk factor; having responsibility for children is an important statistical protector against suicide.

Sickness: Chronic illness is a risk factor.

Although useful for determining a patient's long-term risk for committing suicide, these risk factors are less useful for assessing imminent risk, and imminent risk is the most important factor to assess during a diagnostic interview. While not much research has been done on imminent risk factors, the American Association of Suicidology has agreed on the following short-term warning signs of suicidal behavior (Rudd et al. 2006):

• Rage
• Recklessness
• Feeling trapped
• Increased substance use
• Social withdrawal
• Anxiety/agitation
• Insomnia or hypersomnia
• Mood change
• Lack of purpose or reason for living

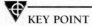
KEY POINT

Suicidality can be a difficult topic to broach, but you must ask about it in every diagnostic interview. Patients are rarely angry or embarrassed about suicidality questions. A majority of depressed patients have at least passing suicidal thoughts from time to time (Winokur 1981), and many patients are relieved when they are asked about suicidality, because it allows them to reveal the true depth of their depression. If they really have not thought about suicide, they will say something like, "Oh no, I could never do anything like that," and will tell you why not.

ASSESSING SUICIDAL IDEATION: INTERVIEW STRATEGIES

Another common disincentive to asking about suicidality is the interviewer's fear of a positive response. You may feel a sense of panic when first confronted with a suicidal patient, but with experience, you will realize that there are degrees of suicidality and that not all suicidal patients require urgent hospitalization.

The CASE Approach

By far, the best method of assessing suicide risk is the CASE approach, which was devised by one of my mentors, Dr. Shawn Shea, and published in his book *The Practical Art of Suicide Assessment* (Shea 2011). I highly recommend that you read this book, as I have, because it provides much more detail regarding his technique and includes innumerable clinical examples.

CASE stands for *Chronological Assessment of Suicidal Events* and will help you to remember to ask about everything relevant to a particular patient's suicidal risk. The technique goes like this:

1. Start by assessing the presenting SI or event.
2. Elicit information about any SI over the past 2 months.
3. Explore past SI.
4. Return to the present and explore any immediate suicidality.

The rationale here is that the process of exploring the presenting event and the past allows you to establish rapport with your patient. This rapport will make it more likely that he or she will be open with you about any imminent suicidal plans, which is really what you most need to assess during the interview.

How does one go about asking the questions required for the CASE approach? Regardless of the time period being explored, the issue of suicidality can be approached in a number of ways. The direct approach can be perfectly acceptable. For example, as part of your evaluation of the SIGECAPS of depression, you can say:

> *Have you felt suicidal?*
> *Have you had thoughts of wanting to hurt yourself?*

 TIP

In some situations, however, this approach may feel jarring to the patient, and a smooth transition may be better:

Sometimes when people feel depressed, they think that they'd be better off dead. Has that thought crossed your mind at all?

Considering all the things you've told me, have you felt so bad that it seems that life is not worth living?

These are both normalizing questions that inquire about "passive" SI. If you get a "yes," you should ask about active SI.

Have you thought about suicide?

What sorts of ways have you thought about to hurt yourself? (Phrased as a behavior expectation.)

Many people with mild to moderate depression endorse passive SI but deny having thought of actually taking some action to harm themselves. This is an important clinical distinction, and you can generally breathe easier if your patient's SI has never gotten beyond the passive stage. If, however, your patient admits to active SI, you'll need to ask an additional series of questions. You want to find out how elaborate and how realistic the suicide plan is.

> *Have you thought about cutting yourself?*
> *Taking an overdose?*
> *Jumping from the window?*

Shooting yourself?
Hanging yourself?

Don't worry that you are putting ideas into their heads. By inquiring specifically about common suicidal behaviors, you are giving patients permission to be truthful and communicating that you're familiar with this difficult topic and won't be put off by a positive answer.

How close have you come to actually hurting yourself?
Have you planned it out in your mind?
Have you acquired any of the things you would need to do something?

Here, you're asking about the presence of a plan and getting a sense of how close the patient has come to carrying out his plan.

Have you actually had the pills in your hand with a glass of water in front of you?
Have you put the pills in your mouth?
What prevented you from actually swallowing them?

This continues specific questioning. The same line of questioning can be used with any other method of suicide the patient may have been fantasizing about.

Do you have a gun in the house?
Do you have access to a rope?
Do you have pills at home?

You should assess how realistic the plan communicated by your patient is. If a patient says he wants to shoot himself, this sounds quite serious, but does he own a gun? If not, does he have access to a friend's or relative's gun? Has he located a shop at which he plans to buy a gun?

Have you written a suicide note?
Have you done anything to put your affairs in order in preparation for your death?

Arrangements such as these are particularly ominous indicators of an imminent suicide attempt.

Are you feeling suicidal right now? Do you have any specific plan to hurt yourself?

Here, you are asking about the immediacy of the intention, so that you can determine the necessity for hospitalization or other urgent intervention.

What has kept you from killing yourself?

This is a very useful topic to introduce. Many desperate patients remain adamantly opposed to suicide for specific reasons, often because they have dependent children or on religious grounds. If you can identify compelling factors that are keeping your patient in the land of the living, reinforce them.

> *If you were to feel more suicidal over the next few days, do you think you could promise to pick up the phone and talk to someone before actually hurting yourself, or would you be in so much pain that you wouldn't want to ask for help?*

TIP

Here, you are trying to discover whether the patient is able to "contract for safety." The whole notion of a safety contract is controversial, and such a contract can certainly provide a false sense of reassurance to the clinician. My feeling is that safety contracts at least do no harm and that they probably have saved lives, because they offer a concrete plan to someone who may be experiencing too much turmoil to think clearly. A good safety contract includes names and numbers of people the patient agrees to contact and a way for her to contact you or your coverage.

ASSESSING HOMICIDAL IDEATION

KEY POINT

Although I have combined the assessment of HI with the assessment of SI, the two are very different creatures. You should assess SI in every patient you interview, but you will ask about HI only in patients you feel are at risk of becoming homicidal. This includes patients in groups who have been identified by researchers as at high risk for homicide (Asnis et al. 1994; Tardiff 1992), such as those who are paranoid, antisocial, or substance abusers or who tell you they are angry at someone in particular.

HI is not the easiest topic to broach during the interview. Interview techniques (see Chapter 4) such as normalization and reduction of guilt are helpful. Once you have introduced the topic, your strategy should be to determine exactly who is the target of the HI and then to assess the seriousness of the ideation. This process is analogous to the assessment of SI, in which you must locate the ideation on a continuum from passive to active to a specific and imminent plan.

CLINICAL VIGNETTE

A 35-year-old woman was admitted to the hospital with the delusion that her mother had been replaced by an impostor who was attempting to take possession of the family home. Knowing that paranoia is a risk factor for HI, the interviewer decided to assess this possibility.

Interviewer: How do you feel about this woman? (Referring to the "impostor" mother.)

Patient: How would you feel? She's taking away all that is mine.

Interviewer: I'd be very angry.

Patient: There you go. I'm being wronged.

Interviewer: I imagine someone in your situation would go to great lengths to prevent this from happening. (Using normalization.)

Patient: I'd say so.

Interviewer: Even to the extent of wanting to do away with that person?

Patient: She's raping my heritage. Death would be too good for her.

Interviewer: It sounds like you'd be happy if she were dead.

Patient: (Looking at interviewer incredulously.) Of course I would.

(At this point, the interviewer has established passive HI; he must now assess whether there is active HI.)

Interviewer: Have you thought about killing her yourself?

Patient: I wish I could. But there are too many others just like her. If I killed her, they would know who did it, and they'd come after me.

Interviewer: So you haven't come up with a plan for killing her?

Patient: Plenty of plans, but where will that get me? I told you, I can't do it.

Interviewer: What sorts of plans?

Patient: The best way would be to cremate her in the house that she wants so much.

Interviewer: You mean set fire to the house?

Patient: It would break my heart to lose the house, but that may be necessary.

The interviewer concluded that the patient was at high risk of following through on her plan to torch her mother's house as a homicide attempt.

This vignette brings up the important issue of what you should do when a patient expresses HI. The Tarasoff decision of 1976 provides guidelines for mental health professionals (Felthous 1991). In essence, you have a responsibility to protect the potential victim. This generally entails informing both the potential victim and the police.

If you do decide to issue a Tarasoff warning, informing your patient of your intentions is a good idea. In such cases, a straightforward approach works best.

> *The law requires me to do what I can to keep this person safe. That means I'm going to try to call him and also call the police.*

You may worry that telling the patient about your intentions will harm the therapeutic alliance. However, according to the only study that actually looked at this issue, in most cases, issuing a warning had either a minimal negative or a positive effect on the alliance (Binder and McNiel 1996).

Assessing Mood Disorders I: Depressive Disorders

Diagnosis of the different types of depressive disorders begins with diagnosis of a major depressive episode (Table 23.1). Once you become an expert at assessing the presence of the NVSs of depression, you will be able to diagnose quickly major depression, atypical depression, seasonal affective disorder (SAD), and dysthymic disorder.

 KEY POINT

It is equally important that you know when *not* to diagnose a depressive disorder. Major depression tends to receive a disproportionate amount of attention in mental health education, partly because it is genuinely common and partly because we are so good at treating it. Nonetheless, you do a disservice to a patient by diagnosing him with major depression if instead he has an adjustment disorder with depressed mood and would benefit more from brief psychotherapy than from medication.

TABLE 23.1. *DSM-5* Criteria for Major Depressive Episode

Five or more of the following symptoms have been present
  for at least 2 wk; at least one of the symptoms is either (a)
  depressed mood or (b) loss of interest or pleasure.
    Depressed mood most of the day, nearly every day
    Markedly diminished interest or pleasure in all, or almost all,
      activities
    Decrease in appetite or significant weight loss
    Insomnia or hypersomnia
    Psychomotor agitation or retardation
    Fatigue or loss of energy
    Feelings of worthlessness or excessive or inappropriate guilt
    Diminished concentration or indecisiveness
    Thoughts of death or SI
    Mnemonic: SIGECAPS

Data from American Psychiatric Association. (2013). *Diagnostic and Statistical Manual of Mental Disorders*, 5th ed. Washington, DC: American Psychiatric Association.

MAJOR DEPRESSIVE EPISODE

Mnemonic: SIGECAPS

A useful mnemonic to guide your questioning of the NVSs of depression is SIGECAPS. It was devised by Dr. Carey Gross at MGH and refers to what one might write on a prescription sheet for a depressed, anergic patient: **SIG**: Energy **CAPS**ules. Each letter refers to one of the major diagnostic criteria for major depressive disorder:

  Sleep disorder (either increased or decreased)*
  Interest deficit (anhedonia)
  Guilt (worthlessness,* *hopelessness,** *regret)*
  Energy deficit*
  Concentration deficit*
  Appetite disorder (either decreased or increased)*
  Psychomotor retardation or agitation
  Suicidality

For dysthymic disorder, two of the six starred symptoms must be present.

Asking About the Symptoms of Depression

The main difficulty for beginning clinicians is in translating the *DSM-5* terminology into language that is meaningful for the patient. A related difficulty is distinguishing true-positive from false-positive responses to questions about symptoms. Most people experience some of the symptoms of major depression to some degree at some time. Establishing that your patient has symptoms severe enough to meet *DSM-5* criteria takes creativity, persistence, and experience.

In this chapter, I discuss techniques for assessing each of the NVSs in turn. First, here are some general tips:

- Establish that the symptom is truly a change from baseline. Many patients may have difficulties with concentration, energy, appetite, and so forth that may be chronic and have little to do with depression. If so, these symptoms cannot "count" toward your diagnosis of a major depressive episode.
- Establish that the symptom has occurred almost every day for 2 weeks. Many patients may react to upsetting events with a few days of NVSs. This does not constitute a major depressive episode, although it may be an adjustment disorder with depressed mood. It's useful to remind patients that you are asking about a specific period.

   Think back carefully: Have you felt depressed pretty much every day over the past 2 weeks?

- Try not to ask leading questions. An example of a leading question is "Has your depression made it hard for you to concentrate?" This implies that decreased concentration would be expected, and a suggestible or malingering patient might answer with a false "yes." An example of a nonleading question would be "Do you think your concentration has been better or worse than normal over the past 2 weeks?" Of course, you can substitute any of the NVSs for "concentration" in this template.

CLINICAL VIGNETTE

An intern was interviewing a 45-year-old nightclub owner. When asked, "How have you been sleeping for the past 2 weeks?" the patient responded, "Terribly. I can't fall asleep before 4 a.m., and then I get up at 10. I'm always tired." The resident considered this statement sufficient to meet criteria for the insomnia of depression, until the patient mentioned that this had been his sleep pattern for the past 6 years and that it had been unchanged over the past 2 weeks. The patient was referred to a sleep clinic and was eventually diagnosed with sleep apnea.

Screening Questions

Are you depressed?

One study showed that this simple question had 100% sensitivity and specificity in diagnosing major depression in the terminally ill, outperforming elaborate screening instruments such as the Beck Depression Inventory (Chochinov et al. 1997).

How has your mood been recently?

This is a nonleading question, but note that it is more specific than asking, "How have you been doing?" or even, "How have you been feeling?" If your patient starts talking about his distress at this point, go to the NVSs of depression. However, if he says "fine," you should move to the more specific question:

Have you ever felt very down or depressed, so depressed that your whole life was affected by it for at least 2 weeks?

SIGECAPS Questions

- Sleep disorder

    Have you been sleeping normally? (A good initial screening question for a sleep problem.)
    What has your sleep pattern been like lately?

(Depending on the adequacy of your patient's response to this question, you may or may not need to follow up with the following questions.)

    What time do you lie down to fall asleep?
    What time do you actually fall asleep?

(To diagnose difficulty falling asleep.)

> *Do you sleep through the night, or do you wake up
> often during the night?*

(To diagnose frequent awakenings.)

> *What time do you usually wake up in the morning?*
> *Do you generally feel rested when you wake up?*
> *Do you feel more or less depressed when you wake up?*
> *How does your mood change as the day goes on?*

(To diagnose early morning awakening and diurnal variation in mood.)

• Interest deficit (anhedonia): Anhedonia is a surprisingly
  difficult symptom to ascertain. Obviously, no patient is
  going to come right out and say, "Doctor, I've been really
  anhedonic lately." You will more likely hear words like,
  "I'm bored all the time," "I have no motivation," or "I
  don't care about anything." One problem is that patients
  may not understand what we mean if we ask, "Can you
  describe your interest level?" or "Have you been taking
  pleasure in things?" A patient may only associate pleasure with extraordinary experiences, such as going on
  vacation, or she may say she has been taking an interest
  in things when in fact her level of interest has decreased
  markedly since the onset of depression. Because of these
  potential pitfalls, it's important to be specific in your
  questioning.

> *Before you felt really sad, what sorts of things would
> you do for fun or for relaxation?*
> *What sorts of hobbies did you have?*
> *Did you read?*
> *Did you play sports or follow the sports teams?*
> *Did you go out to movies?*
> *Did you go out with friends?*

This establishes a baseline against which to compare the
depressed period. You can then go on to ask about how the
depression has affected the patient's activities:

> *Since you have felt depressed, have you noticed that
> you've been any less interested in these pursuits?*
> *Have you found that you've been able to enjoy the
> things that you used to be able to enjoy?*
> *Have you given up doing anything that you normally
> like to do?*

TIP

If the person you are evaluating is already on an antidepressant, particularly if this is a selective serotonin reuptake inhibitor (SSRI), he may seem to have anhedonia, whereas he may actually have "apathy syndrome" secondary to the antidepressant. This occurs in up to 20% to 30% of patients on newer antidepressants and may be caused by lowered levels of brain dopamine.

- Guilt, worthlessness, hopelessness: Here, you want to obtain a sense of how negatively the patient feels about himself. Starting with questions that assess the patient's self-worth often works well:

    How have you been feeling about yourself, in terms of self-esteem, since you've been depressed?
    Do you feel that you are essentially a good person, or do you have your doubts?
    Have you felt especially critical of yourself lately?

These questions touch specifically on the theme of hopelessness:

    How do you see your future?
    Do you have hope that things will get better, or does it look pretty bleak?
    Do you feel helpless to change your situation?

TIP

In assessing guilt, simply asking "Do you feel guilty?" may not be enough, because the patient may not be feeling guilty at that moment, even if she's been feeling guilty frequently over the last few weeks. For this reason, it is helpful to ask about some specific aspects of living that depressed people often feel guilty about.
Have you been feeling guilty or regretful about things that you've done or haven't done? Like not being productive, not reaching your potential, being a burden?

- Energy deficit: Begin with a screening question.

    How has your energy level been over the past couple of weeks?

    If the patient answers "Lousy," make sure that the low energy coincides with the onset of the depression, rather than being a constant feature of her physical state.

    Is this a change for you? Did you feel significantly more energetic before your depression?

- Because medical illness can cause anergia in the absence of depression, you may be misled about the source of the loss of energy, particularly when dealing with patients with chronic medical illnesses or geriatric patients. In such cases, asking about the pattern of energy throughout the day is helpful. Patients with medical illnesses are at their most energetic when they wake up and then feel worse as the day progresses, whereas depressed patients often wake up feeling low and anergic and feel better later in the day.
- Concentration deficit.

    Have you been able to focus on things well? How has your concentration been?

    (These general questions are sometimes sufficient for screening purposes.)

    Have you felt more absentminded than usual?
    Have you noticed any changes in your memory?

    (These get at the pseudodementia sometimes seen in depression.)

    Have you had problems making decisions?

    Sometimes, the first sign of concentration problems is difficulty in making basic decisions such as "What should I make for dinner?" or "Should I go out tonight or not?"

    If you were to sit down with a newspaper in front of you, would you be able to read an entire article from start to finish without losing your concentration, or do you have to read the same sentence over and over again?
    Can you watch a half-hour television show from start to finish without losing your focus?
    Have you noticed that you haven't been able to get quite as much done at work as before?

Concentration questions such as these can be tailored to the patient, depending on what sorts of activities he normally engages in. One study of 31 depressed patients found that the activities most commonly reported to be impaired were television watching (71%), reading (68%), and household jobs (65%) (Pilowsky and Boulton 1970).

KEY POINT

We are often taught to look mainly for loss of appetite and consequent weight loss in depression, with the exceptions of atypical depression and SAD. However, studies show that weight gain is quite common in typical major depression as well (Stunkard et al. 1990; Weissenburger et al. 1986). In one study of 93 patients with typical depression, 37% gained weight, 32% lost weight, and 31% showed no change in weight (Weissenburger et al. 1986), so you'll want to make sure to phrase your appetite question in a nonleading way.

* Appetite

    Since you've been depressed, have you noticed that your appetite has increased, decreased, or stayed about the same?
    Have you lost or gained weight since you've been depressed?
    Do your clothes fit you differently?
    How many meals a day do you eat?

These questions often lead to more accurate information; you can quantitate how much the patient is actually eating, and the patient may in fact be surprised to realize that he has been eating less or more than usual.

    Does food taste good to you?

Depressed patients sometimes identify their eating problem not so much as a decrease in appetite, but as a sense that food has become tasteless and unenjoyable, "like cardboard," as one patient told me.

TIP

This part of the interview provides a natural transition for asking about symptoms of eating disorders. For example, if a patient tells you that she overeats when depressed, ask if she binges and purges as well (see Chapter 29).

• Psychomotor agitation and retardation: Although the *DSM-5* specifies that psychomotor agitation and retardation should be diagnosed based on what you observe in the patient during the evaluation, the following questions may also be helpful:

> *Sometimes when people get depressed, they notice that their movements really slow down, almost as though their limbs are made of lead. Has that happened to you? (For psychomotor retardation.)*
> *Have you been more restless than usual? Have you been pacing, wringing your hands, unable to sit down for long? (For psychomotor agitation.)*

• Suicidality (see Chapter 22)

OTHER DEPRESSIVE SYNDROMES

Persistent Depressive Disorder (Dysthymia)

Mnemonic: ACHEWS. Two of these six, with depressed mood, for 2 years are indicative of persistent depressive disorder, which in DSM-IV was called "dysthymia."

Appetite disorder (either decreased or increased appetite)
Concentration deficit
Hopelessness
Energy deficit
Worthlessness (low self-esteem)
Sleep disorder (either increased or decreased sleep)

The persistently depressed patient is "allergic" to happiness; hence, the mnemonic refers to a patient's (misspelled) sneezes (achoos), brought on by exposure to happiness. To meet the criteria, the patient must have 2 years of depressed mood, along with two of the six symptoms in the list.

Persistent depressive disorder (PDD) is often diagnosed early in the interview in the context of the chief complaint. When a patient presents with symptoms of depression, a good screening question for PDD is

> *When was the last time you remember not feeling depressed?*

The typical PDD patient will answer "many years." In fact, the average duration of the disorder is 16 years (Klein et al. 1993).

Along with depressed mood, you also have to establish the continuous presence of at least two of the ACHEWS symptoms for 2 years or more. The most efficient way to do this is to start with depressive symptoms that your patient has already mentioned, rather than going through your list. Thus, if you have already heard about her lethargy, ask about that:

> *Over these last 2 years, in which you say you've been depressed, has your energy been low most of the time?*

Atypical Depression

Atypical depression is a depressive subtype characterized by "reverse" NVSs (e.g., *increased* appetite rather than anorexia and *increased* need for sleep rather than insomnia), mood reactivity (the ability to be cheered up by positive events), a pattern of rejection sensitivity throughout one's adult life, and a feeling of being weighed down ("leaden paralysis").

Research has cast doubt on the validity of this diagnosis (Lam and Stewart 1996), but it's still worth asking about it because patients with these features probably respond particularly well to MAOI antidepressants.

Seasonal Affective Disorder

Once you have established that the patient has episodes of major depression, ask if these episodes follow any seasonal pattern. The most common pattern is depression in the winter and euthymia in the summer.

> *Have you noticed that your depressions consistently
> come on or get worse in the winter and then go away
> when the weather improves?*

SAD is similar to atypical depression in that reverse NVSs
are usually present, such as carbohydrate craving (with consequent weight gain) and hypersomnia.

If your patient is having a hard time remembering a seasonal aspect to the depression, you can jog his memory by
asking

> *Do you generally go on vacation to a sunny place dur-
> ing the winter? Do you find that your mood dramati-
> cally improves during the vacation?*

Obviously, anybody's mood improves to some extent during vacation, but the patient with SAD will report a more
extreme mood shift that often lasts for several weeks after his
return, with a gradual lapsing back into depression thereafter.
This mimics the response to light therapy.

Assessing Mood Disorders II: Bipolar Disorder

Essential Concepts
Screening Questions
- Have you ever had a period of a week or so when you felt so happy and energetic that you didn't need to sleep and your friends told you that you were talking too fast or that you were behaving differently and strangely?
- Have you had periods when you were snapping at people and getting into arguments?

Mnemonic: **DIGFAST**
Recommended time: 1 minute if negative screen; 5 minutes if positive screen.

MANIC EPISODE

Bipolar disorder tends to be under diagnosed by beginning clinicians. Most patients who present for psychiatric interviews appear demoralized, depressed, or anxious, and one isn't intuitively moved to ask about periods of extreme happiness. It's helpful to realize that bipolar disorder usually presents first as a major depression and that up to 20% of patients with depression go on to develop bipolar disorder (Blacker and Tsuang 1992).

Even when you *do* remember to ask about mania, there is another roadblock: a high rate of false-positive responses. Many patients report periods of euphoria and high energy that represent normal variations in mood rather than mania. Thus, the most effective screening questions for mania ask about other people's perceptions as well as the patient's self-perception.

In general, you should keep referring to a particular period as you ask your questions, because many people experience

TABLE 24.1. DSM-5 Criteria for Manic Episode

1. A distinct period of abnormally and persistently elevated, expansive, or irritable mood, lasting at least 1 wk, or such a mood of any duration if hospitalization is necessary.
2. Persistence of three or more of the following symptoms (four if the mood is only irritable) during the period of mood disturbance:

   Mnemonic: **DIGFAST**

   Distractibility

   Indiscretion (excessive involvement in pleasurable activities that have a high potential for painful consequences)

   Grandiosity or inflated self-esteem

   Flight of ideas or racing thoughts

   Activity increase (increase in goal-directed activity or psychomotor agitation)

   Sleep deficit

   Talkativeness (pressured speech)

Data from American Psychiatric Association. (2013). *Diagnostic and Statistical Manual of Mental Disorders*, 5th ed. Washington, DC: American Psychiatric Association.

the separate diagnostic criteria of mania at various points in their lives (e.g., spending foolishly, talking unusually fast, being unusually distractible), but unless a number of these symptoms have co-occurred during a discrete period (at least 1 week or 4 days for hypomania), a manic episode cannot be diagnosed (Table 24.1).

Screening Questions

> *Have you ever had a period of a week or so when you felt so happy and energetic that you didn't need to sleep and your friends told you that you were talking too fast or that you were behaving differently and strangely?*

If you get a "yes" here, find out when that period was and how long it lasted, and then continually refer to that period when you ask about the diagnostic criteria for mania. If the patient cannot remember such a period lasting an entire week, you should suspect that mania is not the diagnosis. Determine the circumstances of the elevated mood. Being really happy for a couple of days after college graduation, for example, is not mania.

Has there been a time when you felt just the opposite of depressed, so that for a week or so you felt as if you were on an adrenaline high and could conquer the world?

The preceding question about mania is handy if you have just finished asking about symptoms of depression.

Do you experience wild mood swings in which you feel incredibly good for a week or more and then crash down into a depression?

Interpret responses to this question cautiously, because some patients who respond with an emphatic "yes" are referring to recurrent episodes of depression without mania or hypomania.

Have you had periods when you were snapping at people all the time and getting into arguments with them?

This gets at the diagnosis of irritable, mixed, or dysphoric mania. Obviously, false-positive responses abound here, and following up with questions establishing that this period of irritability represented a manic episode, rather than a depression or simply a transient foul mood, will be no small task.

Has anyone ever said that you were manic or that you had bipolar disorder?

If someone answers "yes" to this, pay close attention. It's not common for healthy people to have been called *manic* by someone.

Use DIGFAST to Elicit Diagnostic Criteria

The author of the DIGFAST jewel is unknown, but it's very useful in remembering the diagnostic criteria for a manic episode. The term apparently refers to the speed with which a manic patient would dig a hole if put to the task.

Mnemonic: **DIGFAST**

Distractibility
Indiscretion (DSM-5's "excessive involvement in pleasurable activities")
Grandiosity
Flight of ideas
Activity increase
Sleep deficit (decreased need for sleep)
Talkativeness (pressured speech)

In addition to expansive mood, the patient must qualify for three of the seven DIGFAST symptoms, or four of seven if the primary mood is irritable.

When you ask about the symptoms of mania, precede your questions with something such as, "During the period last year when you felt high, were you ...?" This way, you can ensure that all the symptoms have occurred within the same time frame.

TIP

Be sure to ask whether these behaviors occurred in the context of alcohol or drug abuse. If so, you'll have to judge whether the manic behavior is actually secondary to a substance abuse problem or whether the substance abuse is secondary to mania. This is often a difficult question to sort out.

Distractibility

Were you having trouble thinking? Was this because things around you would get you off track?

KEY POINT

Remember that the distractibility of a patient with mania is different from the decreased concentration of a depressed person. A person with mania is distractible not because his thinking is slowed down, but because his mind is working so quickly and furiously that any mental stimulus, internal or external, knocks him off track.

Indiscretion

During the period we've been talking about, how did you spend your time?
Were you doing things that were out of character or unusual for you?

These are nice questions to start with, because they are relatively unbiased and unlikely to lead the patient to invalid responses.

> *Were you doing things that caused trouble for you or your family?*

This is a good question because it doesn't imply a judgment of the morality of any particular behavior—it merely asks if a behavior has caused trouble for anyone.

> *Were you doing things that showed a lack of judgment, such as driving too quickly, running red lights, or spending too much money?*
> *Did you do anything sexual during this period that was unusual for you?*

KEY POINT

Although you risk pushing a patient's "being judged" button with these questions, most patients respond straightforwardly, especially if the rapport is good. One potential pitfall is assuming that any period of increased spending is diagnostic of a manic episode. In fact, some patients have periods of compulsive buying without mania; such buying may be motivated by a need to reduce feelings of depression or anxiety (Lejoyeux et al. 1997).

Grandiosity

> *During this period, did you feel especially self-confident, as if you could conquer the world?*
> *Did you have particularly good ideas?*
> *Did you feel that you were right and that everybody else was wrong?*

Often, this is a good opportunity to elicit the grandiose delusions that are so common in mania:

> *Did you feel like you had any special powers?*
> *Did you feel more religious than normal?*

Flight of Ideas

> *Did you have so many ideas that you could barely keep up with them?*
> *Were thoughts racing through your head?*
> *Were other people having a hard time understanding your ideas?*

When assessing flight of ideas, be aware that "racing thoughts" per se are not specific to bipolar disorder. Patients with anxiety disorders, ADHD, or depression with anxious ruminations commonly describe their thoughts as "racing." A good way to distinguish manic racing from anxious racing is to ask:

> *Were your thoughts racing in a good way or in an unpleasant, worried, or depressed way?*

Patients experiencing manic episodes often have a sense of an "accelerated" thought process that is like a joyride in a stolen car. Patients with anxiety or depression will feel very differently.

Activity Increase

The activity increase criterion is similar to indiscretion but focuses specifically on the frenetic nature of the activity.

> *Were you more active than usual?*
> *Were you constantly starting new projects or hobbies?*
> *Did you have so much energy that you felt it was hard to calm down?*

Sleep Deficit

> *Did you need less sleep than usual?*
> *Did you ever stay up all night doing all kinds of things, such as working on projects or calling people?*

TIP

Be careful not to confuse the sleeplessness of depression or anxiety with mania. Patients with mania stay awake because they have so much to think about and do, whereas depressed patients stay awake because they feel tortured by their feelings. Therefore, be sure to ask patients what sorts of things they do when they can't sleep. Patients with mania will report productive activities, whereas depressed patients will read or watch television as they wait for the solace of sleep.

Talkativeness

> *Did you find it hard to stop talking?*
> *Did other people tell you that they had trouble under-standing you?*
> *Did friends have to interrupt you to get a word in edgewise?*
> *Were you using the phone more than usual?*

Other Tips for Diagnosing Mania

- **History of hospitalization:** If a patient was hospitalized during a "hyper" period, chances are good that this was indeed a manic episode.
- **Interview with relatives and friends:** One of the hallmarks of mania is a lack of insight, making verification of historical information particularly important.
- **Family history of bipolar disorder:** Bipolar disorder is one of the most inheritable of all psychiatric disorders (see Chapter 17).

BIPOLAR DISORDER, TYPE II: THE HYPOMANIC EPISODE

In bipolar disorder, type II, patients have a history of depressive and hypomanic episodes. Hypomania can be hard to diagnose (Table 24.2). Essentially, it amounts to a psychiatric diagnosis for exuberant and often very productive happiness. However, patients with bipolar II spend much of their nonhypomanic time in depression, which is why bipolar II is important not to miss. Use the same DIGFAST questions

TABLE 24.2. DSM-5 Criteria for Hypomanic Episode

Same as the criteria for manic episode except that:
1. The period of expansive or irritable mood needs to last only 4 d rather than a full week.
2. The episode is not severe enough to cause "marked impairment in social or occupational functioning."

Data from American Psychiatric Association. (2013). *Diagnostic and Statistical Manual of Mental Disorders*, 5th ed. Washington, DC: American Psychiatric Association.

to diagnose hypomania that are used to diagnose mania. The patient with hypomania will describe definite high periods that have not caused real problems in her life. When hypomanic periods alternate with depressed periods, the proper diagnosis is *bipolar, type II disorder*.

Assessing Anxiety, Obsessive, and Trauma Disorders

Anxiety is a common symptom and can be a frustrating diagnostic issue for beginning interviewers because of the enormous number of disorders that can present with anxiety. For example, many patients with major depression, mania, and schizophrenia also report significant anxiety, even in the absence of a specific anxiety disorder (Brown et al. 2001).

Nonetheless, it is important to be systematic about diagnosing anxiety disorders, particularly because many disorder-specific psychotherapies have been developed. For example, the cognitive-behavioral approach to the treatment of panic disorder is very different from the cognitive-behavioral approach to social phobia (Barlow 2014).

You should develop a systematic approach to asking about the major *DSM-5* anxiety disorders, in addition to OCD and PTSD (*DSM-5* removed the latter two disorders from its anxiety section, but I believe they are still most usefully considered disorders of fear/anxiety).

1. Panic disorder
2. Agoraphobia
3. GAD
4. Social anxiety disorder
5. Specific phobia
6. OCD
7. PTSD

Even if you ask all the right questions, distinguishing among some of these disorders, especially the first four, can be tricky. A useful aid is the *DSM-5 Handbook of Differential Diagnosis* (First 2013), which contains excellent tables to guide you in differentiating one disorder from another.

Following are suggested questions for diagnosing the anxiety disorders, along with brief reminders of the diagnostic criteria for each disorder.

PANIC DISORDER

The first step in diagnosing panic disorder is establishing that your patient has had panic attacks. Remember, however, that a panic attack does not imply panic disorder. In fact, ~35% of healthy people report having had a panic attack within the past year (Norton et al. 1986), whereas only 4.7% of the population will ever develop full-blown panic disorder (Kessler et al. 2005). Panic attacks are often responses to specific situations that people can successfully avoid (e.g., claustrophobia, specific phobias). Panic may signal a disorder other than panic disorder, such as social phobia or PTSD. Finally, many people experience panic and anxiety that are not quite severe enough to meet criteria for a *DSM-5* disorder (Table 25.1).

The initial screening question for panic is straightforward:

> *Have you ever had a panic or anxiety attack?*

Most people have heard the term *panic attack*. However, a positive response to this question requires verification, because many people define a subpanic level of anxiety as a panic attack. This seems especially true of patients with GAD. Such patients may respond, "I'm always having a panic

TABLE 25.1. DSM-5 Criteria for Panic Disorder

1. Recurrent unexpected panic attacks (must have 4 of 13 symptoms): mnemonic for panic attack, Heart, Breathlessness, Fear
   Heart cluster: palpitations, chest pain, nausea
   Breathlessness cluster: shortness of breath, choking sensation, dizziness, paresthesias, hot/cold waves
   Fear cluster: fear of dying, fear of going crazy, sweating, shaking, derealization/depersonalization
2. At least one of the attacks has been followed by 1 mo (or more) of at least one of the following three:
   Fear of another attack occurring
   Persistent worry about the implications or consequences of the attack
   A significant change in behavior because of the attacks

Data from American Psychiatric Association. (2013). *Diagnostic and Statistical Manual of Mental Disorders*, 5th ed. Washington, DC: American Psychiatric Association.

attack. I'm having one right now." Other patients will ask you what you mean by a panic attack. You need to provide a good definition in lay terms to effectively diagnose panic attack:

> *A panic attack is a sudden rush of fear and nervousness in which your heart pounds, you get short of breath, and you're afraid you're going to lose control or even die. Has that ever happened to you?*

In my experience, this question is highly sensitive and specific for diagnosing true panic attack. Patients who hear this definition and say unequivocally, "Oh no, I've been nervous before, but I've never had anything like that," are unlikely to have ever had a panic attack. For patients who answer "yes," ask them to describe the experience:

> *When did you last have one of these attacks? Can you describe that attack for me? What were you doing when it started? How did it make you feel, and how long did it last?*

The best way to assess the clinical significance of a panic attack is to listen to your patient describe one. You will find out which anxiety symptoms are present and whether the attacks have a specific precipitant.

> *When you have these attacks, do you notice any of the*
> *following symptoms: sweating, shaking, tingling in*
> *your hands or lips, shortness of breath, choking, your*
> *heart pounding, chest pain, nausea, or a feeling that*
> *you're about to die or go crazy?*

Although I've listed all these symptoms in one paragraph for convenience, you should ask about them one by one to give your patient time to think about each. Use the symptom cluster technique (heart, breathlessness, fear) to remember each of the symptoms.

> *When you have a panic attack, does it come out of*
> *the blue, or do you pretty much know what's going*
> *to cause it?*

Remember that to meet criteria for panic disorder, the panic attacks have to be unexpected (i.e., out of the blue). Otherwise, panic attacks may signify social phobia, if the trigger is a social situation; PTSD, if the trigger is a flashback; agoraphobia, if the trigger is a hard-to-escape place; or a specific phobia with a variety of possible triggers.

> *Has one of these attacks ever woken you up at night?*
> *Do you remember when you had your first panic*
> *attack?*

These two questions will increase the specificity of your exploration. If a patient is awakened at night by panic, it's very likely a true, unexpected panic attack. (Some clinicians would also wonder about a history of sexual abuse.) In addition, people with true panic disorders often distinctly remember their first panic attack.

Beyond simply establishing the bare bones of the diagnosis, you should make some attempt to assess whether the patient might be a good candidate for cognitive-behavioral therapy (CBT). In many cases, CBT works better than medication for panic disorder, particular over the long haul (Barlow et al. 2000). Patients who will respond well to CBT are those who can identify "catastrophic cognition" in response to the panic sensations. A typical interchange follows:

Interviewer: When you have panic attacks, what exactly goes through your mind?
Patient: I think I'm going to pass out, or worse.
Interviewer: Do you think you're going to die?

Patient: Yes, that's when I really get scared.
Interviewer: You mean the panic sensations become more intense when you have those thoughts?
Patient: Definitely.
Interviewer: But have you ever actually passed out?
Patient: No.
Interviewer: Do you think it's possible that your thought process makes you feel even more anxious than you'd otherwise feel?
Patient: I never thought about it that way, but I guess you're right.

Such a patient would likely be a good prospect for referral to a cognitive-behavioral therapist after you have finished your diagnostic interview.

AGORAPHOBIA

Agoraphobia (Table 25.2) often develops as a complication of panic disorder, thought it can be a free-standing disorder (American Psychiatric Association 2013). Usually, the patient has a few panic attacks and gradually begins to avoid situations that he associates with those attacks, a process termed *phobic avoidance*. The agoraphobic avoids situations in which a quick escape would be difficult. Typical examples include crowded places (e.g., restaurants, stores, trains, buses) and driving a car, especially in heavy traffic or far from home.

> *Have you started to avoid things because of your panic attacks?*

Ask this question of every patient with panic disorder. Agoraphobia accompanies panic disorder so commonly that the *DSM*-III-R describes no diagnosis of agoraphobia without panic disorder.

TABLE 25.2. DSM-5 Criteria for Agoraphobia

1. Anxiety about being in places or situations from which escape might be difficult or embarrassing
2. Situations are avoided or are endured with marked distress

Data from American Psychiatric Association. (2013). *Diagnostic and Statistical Manual of Mental Disorders*, 5th ed. Washington, DC: American Psychiatric Association.

> *Do you have problems with crowds? Buses or subways?*
> *Restaurants? Bridges? Driving places?*

Be sure not to confuse agoraphobia, a generalized fear of a variety of situations in which escape might be difficult, with a specific phobia of bridges or buses or with PTSD, in which a specific situation reminiscent of a past trauma may provoke a fear response.

> *Do you get anxious when you leave home?*

At its worst, the agoraphobic's world constricts so much that leaving the home is a terrifying prospect.

GENERALIZED ANXIETY DISORDER

The patient with GAD is the prototypical worrier, who worries about several things for months on end and is incapable of relaxing.

Begin with this screening question:

> *Are you a worrier?*

Like the screening question for panic disorder, this question is exceedingly unlikely to elicit a "no" answer from someone who truly has GAD.

> *What do you worry about?*

Common topics of generalized anxiety include the health of relatives (especially children), the quality of a romantic relationship, job or school performance, and the possibility that possessions will break down or be stolen. However, certain topics of worry suggest other diagnoses. For example, excessive worry about performance in social situations may indicate social phobia, worry about having a panic attack suggests panic disorder, and excessive worry about bodily sensations points to somatization disorder. Don't make the mistake of overdiagnosing GAD when the actual diagnosis is something more specific.

On the other hand, some patients experience free-floating anxiety without having a particular focus for their worries. Such patients do not meet criteria for GAD or any other anxiety disorder; diagnostic possibilities to consider include

TABLE 25.3. DSM-5 Criteria for GAD

1. Excessive anxiety and worry, occurring more days than not for at least 6 mo, about a number of events or activities
2. Difficulty controlling the worry
3. Anxiety associated with at least three of the following six symptoms: mnemonic, **M**acbeth **F**rets **C**onstantly **R**egarding **I**llicit **S**ins
   Muscle tension
   Fatigue
   Concentration difficulty
   Restlessness or feeling on edge
   Irritability
   Sleep disturbance

Data from American Psychiatric Association. (2013). *Diagnostic and Statistical Manual of Mental Disorders*, 5th ed. Washington, DC: American Psychiatric Association.

major depression, schizophrenia, or a medication side effect such as akathisia (i.e., a feeling of restlessness caused by antipsychotic medication).

> *Over these past few months of worrying, have you noticed that you've been feeling jittery? Irritable? Do you feel tension in your muscles? Do you tire easily? Do you have insomnia? Do you have problems concentrating?*

The *DSM-5* requires that GAD patients experience at least three of the preceding six NVSs (Table 25.3). Otherwise, too many quite happy and functional worriers would be receiving psychiatric diagnoses.

SOCIAL ANXIETY DISORDER

The person with social phobia fears embarrassment and humiliation in a range of different public situations, such as public speaking, meeting someone new, or eating in front of others. All of us fear some of these things to some extent, but the social phobic's fear is unusually intense, to the point of having a panic attack (Table 25.4). Social phobics will often give you a clue to their condition by being shy and awkward during the interview, avoiding eye contact, and laughing nervously.

TABLE 25.4. DSM-5 Criteria for Social Phobia

1. A fear of social performance situations in which the person is exposed to unfamiliar people or to possible scrutiny by others
2. Exposure to the feared situation almost invariably provokes anxiety, which may take the form of a panic attack

Data from American Psychiatric Association. (2013). *Diagnostic and Statistical Manual of Mental Disorders*, 5th ed. Washington, DC: American Psychiatric Association.

The screening question is

Are you uncomfortable in social situations?

You may need to specify the situations you have in mind:

I mean situations such as public speaking, asking questions in front of a class, or being at a party or in a meeting.

If you get a "yes" to the screening question, ask

How uncomfortable do you get? Do you get to the point of having a panic attack?
Is this anxiety so intolerable that you would go out of your way to avoid any social situations?

SPECIFIC PHOBIA

A specific phobia is easily diagnosed with the questions

Do you have any special fears, such as a fear of insects or a fear of flying?
Have you ever had a panic attack when you've been around this thing that you fear?

If you get positive responses to these questions, you must further establish that the specific phobia interferes significantly with psychosocial functioning (Table 25.5).

TABLE 25.5. DSM-5 Criteria for Specific Phobia

1. Excessive and unreasonable fear of a specific object or situation
2. Exposure to the phobic stimulus causes intense anxiety

Data from American Psychiatric Association. (2013). *Diagnostic and Statistical Manual of Mental Disorders*, 5th ed. Washington, DC: American Psychiatric Association.

OBSESSIVE-COMPULSIVE DISORDER

OCD is a commonly overlooked diagnosis because patients rarely volunteer such embarrassing symptoms without being asked. Thus, including OCD questions as part of your routine PROS is particularly important.

Begin with the following high-yield screening question:

> *Do you have symptoms of an obsessive-compulsive disorder, such as needing to wash your hands all the time because you feel dirty, constantly checking things, or having annoying thoughts pop into your head over and over?*

Although this may sound like an excessively long question, so much information is packed into it that if you get a flatly confident "no" in response, you are unlikely to find OCD by digging further. A "yes" requires further probing, because patients will often say that they check or wash, but on detailed questioning, they may not meet criteria for OCD (Table 25.6).

For example, if a patient says that he checks things, you must establish that he is uncomfortably *driven* to do so:

TABLE 25.6. DSM-5 Criteria for OCD

Mnemonic: **W**ashing and **S**traightening **M**ake **C**lean **H**ouses
Washing
Straightening
Mental rituals (e.g., magical words, numbers)
Checking
Hoarding
Must have either obsessions or compulsions
Obsessions
Recurrent intrusive thoughts
Impulses
Images that cause anxiety and that the person tries to ignore or suppress
Compulsions
Repeated behaviors or mental acts that the person feels driven to perform in response to an obsession
Behaviors or acts aimed at preventing or reducing distress

Data from American Psychiatric Association. (2013). *Diagnostic and Statistical Manual of Mental Disorders*, 5th ed. Washington, DC: American Psychiatric Association.

> *When you check to make sure the door is locked, do*
> *you feel like you really have to check it, and that if you*
> *didn't you'd feel very uncomfortable?*

You must establish that the checking takes up enough of a person's time to significantly interfere with day-to-day activities:

> *How many times do you check the door usually? Is it*
> *just once or twice or do you have to check it 10 or 20*
> *times to be satisfied that it's locked?*

Patients may present with a number of different types of obsessions and compulsions. You can often ask about obsessions and compulsions in the same question:

> *Do you wash your hands excessively because of wor-*
> *ries about dirt or germs?*
> *Do you feel the need to check things around the house*
> *because of a fear that bad things might happen if you*
> *don't?*
> *Do you feel the need to save every little scrap of paper*
> *because of a fear that you'll need them all sometime?*

For mental rituals, ask

> *Do you often find yourself counting things or naming*
> *things for no particular reason?*

To determine the degree of functional impairment caused by the symptoms, you can ask

> *How much time do you usually need to get ready to*
> *leave the house in the morning?*

A patient with many cleaning and dressing rituals may take 2 to 3 hours or more to get showered and dressed.

POSTTRAUMATIC STRESS DISORDER

Because most people have heard of PTSD, the screening question can include the term, along with a brief definition.

> *Do you have posttraumatic stress disorder, which*
> *means having memories or dreams of a terrible expe-*
> *rience, like being attacked by someone or surviving a*
> *natural disaster?*

Researchers have found that listing examples of traumatic events increases patient recall in PTSD (Solomon and Davidson 1997). If your patient answers "no" to such questions, PTSD is unlikely. A positive response requires that you establish the presence of the *DSM-5* criteria (Table 25.7).

What sort of experience was it?

Asking in this general manner, rather than inquiring directly about the experience, gives your patient permission to answer vaguely, which may be all she can tolerate. Remember that a hallmark of PTSD is the need to avoid the memory of the trauma; allow your patient to do this if she needs to.

Once you have established that a traumatic experience occurred, ask about each of the criteria.

* Reexperience (**R**emembers)

    Does the experience come back to haunt you from time to time?
    Have you had nightmares or flashbacks of this experience?

TABLE 25.7. DSM-5 Criteria for Posttraumatic Stress Disorder

Mnemonic: **R**emembers **A**trocious **N**uclear **A**ttacks
1. The person has experienced a traumatic event that involved actual or threatened death or a threat to the physical integrity of self or others.
2. The traumatic event is persistently **R**eexperienced via memories, dreams, flashbacks, or intense distress when the person is exposed to events that are symbolic of the original event.
3. Stimuli associated with the event are persistently **A**voided, for example, avoiding certain activities or thoughts, amnesia for the event.
4. The person experiences **N**egative cognitions and feelings, as in negative beliefs about oneself or the world, inability to have positive emotions, diminished interest in various activities, or a sense of foreshortened future.
5. Increased **A**rousal occurs: sleep disturbance, irritability, difficulty concentrating, hypervigilance, exaggerated startle response.
6. The disturbance lasts at least 1 month.

Data from American Psychiatric Association. (2013). *Diagnostic and Statistical Manual of Mental Disorders*, 5th ed. Washington, DC: American Psychiatric Association.

If your patient doesn't understand what you mean by *flash-backs,* you can elaborate:

> *Do you find that you're remembering the event and you truly feel like you're back there again?*

- Avoidance (Atrocious)

> *Do you find yourself avoiding things that you associate with the memory?*

Inquiring about specific activities or situations related to the actual trauma is better than using this general question. For example, if the trauma was a rape, you might ask

> *Do you find yourself avoiding going out with men to avoid remembering what happened?*

If the experience was an automobile accident, you might ask

> *Do you avoid driving or even getting into cars because of that experience?*

- Negativity (Nuclear): In DSM-IV, this criterion was called "numbing." DSM-5 broadened it to include not just symptoms of numbing but other kinds of emotional or cognitive negativity. Many are similar to symptoms of depression, especially anhedonia and decreased energy. You may have asked about them earlier in the interview. Others relate to a more general sense of unhappiness (such as fear, anger, and shame) or a general negative view of oneself and the world.

> *Since the trauma, has your interest in life gone downhill?*

Your patient may describe a diminished range of activities.

> *Have friendships suffered? Has it been harder to have feelings for loved ones?*
> *Has your sense of the future changed?*

A PTSD patient may respond with "I don't see any future" or "I don't even think about the future."

> *Do you think the world in general is a good place or a bad place?*

While simplistic, this question is good at opening people up to a discussion of how the trauma has affected the way they see the world.

- Arousal (Attacks): As in numbing, many symptoms of hyperarousal are also typical symptoms of major depression, such as insomnia, difficulty concentrating, and irritability. Hypervigilance and a startle response are more specific to PTSD.

  Since the trauma, have you felt hyper and on edge much of the time?
  Do you startle easily?

Assessing Alcohol Use Disorder

> **Essential Concepts**
> * Do you enjoy a drink now and then?
> * Ask CAGE questions.
> * Do you use any recreational drugs, such as marijuana, LSD, or cocaine?
>
> *Recommended time:* 2 minutes for screening; 5 to 10 minutes for probing, if screen is positive.

> *First you take a drink, then the drink takes a drink, then the drink takes you.*
>
> F. Scott Fitzgerald

In an initial diagnostic interview, you will probably not have time to do a complete assessment of the history, extent, and consequences of a patient's substance abuse problem. Such an assessment requires a full session in itself. What, then, are your more limited goals? There are three:

1. Determine whether your patient meets DSM-5 criteria for alcohol/drug use disorder.
2. Get a sense of the severity of the problem.
3. Determine how the alcohol use interacts with any comorbid psychiatric disorders present.

The most important tip for beginners is to be **nonjudgmental**. This requires some soul-searching because most of us have negative prejudices about substance abusers, and we tend to see them as being morally suspect. Be aware of the extent to which you hold such attitudes, and evaluate whether they are accurate. Try to meet with recovered alcoholics. Their stories are often poignant and will help you to develop a more sympathetic and compassionate attitude. Learn about the disease model of alcoholism (Vaillant 1995). The more you can view alcoholism as similar to the other psychiatric disorders you treat, the fewer prejudices you will retain.

ASSESSMENT TECHNIQUES

Screening Questions

 TIP

The best quick screen for alcoholism remains the tried-and-true CAGE questionnaire (see below; Ewing 1984), in which a positive response to two or more of the items implies a 95% chance of alcohol abuse or dependence. However, one study (Steinweg and Worth 1993) suggests that the way interviewers transition to the CAGE questions profoundly affects the questionnaire's sensitivity. Researchers divided 43 confirmed alcoholics into two groups. In group I, the CAGE was introduced with an open-ended question, such as "Do you have a drink now and then?" In group II, patients were first asked to quantitate their alcohol intake with the question, "How much do you drink?" Sensitivity toward the CAGE questions was dramatically higher in group I (95%) than in group II (32%), demonstrating the importance of beginning the screening in a nonjudgmental way.

CAGE questionnaire:

Cut down: "Have you felt you should cut down on your drinking?"

Annoyed: "Have people annoyed you by getting on your case about your drinking?"

Guilty: "Have you ever felt bad or guilty about your drinking?"

Eye-opener: "Have you ever needed to take a drink first thing in the morning to steady your nerves or get rid of a hangover?"

Begin your screen with the nonthreatening question:

Do you enjoy a drink now and then?

If a patient answers, "I never drink," you should ask, "Why not?" Most people of the American culture have a drink occasionally; people who make a point of not drinking are uncommon. They may avoid drinking because they are recovered alcoholics, because they have a family member with a serious drinking problem, or for religious or ethical reasons. Most people will answer with something like, "Oh, I have glass of wine with dinner" or "I have a beer when I barbecue."

 TIP

Kevin Rice, LCSW, says that "When asking about substance abuse, I find that the word 'experiment' almost always elicits a more accurate response than the word 'use.' An inquiry into the possible use or abuse of marijuana would begin, 'Have you ever experimented with marijuana?'" (Shea 2007).

Once you have ascertained any use of alcohol of other substances, jump right into the CAGE questions:

Cut down: Have you ever tried to cut down on your drinking?

A cardinal feature of alcoholism is the loss of control over drinking, and this question gets at that issue. If the patient answers "yes," follow up with

What made you decide to cut down?

The answer to this question will likely move you into an exploration of the adverse consequences of drinking that the patient experienced. (See next section.)

Annoyed: Have you ever been annoyed about friends' or family's criticism of your drinking?

The severe alcoholic will not only have been criticized by loved ones for his drinking but may have completely alienated most important people in his life.

Guilty: Have you ever felt a little guilty about your drinking?

Again, a positive response is an invitation to further exploration.

Eye-opener: Have you ever felt hungover or shaky in the morning and taken a drink to get rid of that feeling?

This behavior is a good indicator of out-of-control drinking.

As your final screening question, ask matter-of-factly:

Do you think that you have a drinking problem?

I have been amazed at how many patients answer "no" to all the CAGE questions and then answer "yes" to this one.

If the patient has answered "no" to the CAGE questions and the drinking problem question, and if there were no clues to a drinking problem (e.g., the odor of alcohol on the breath), the patient has no drinking problem, and you can ask the general question:

> *Do you use any recreational drugs, like marijuana, LSD, or cocaine?*

If the patient gives a negative answer to this question, you can move out of the substance abuse area.

 TIP

If a patient has admitted to a drinking problem, I have found it useful to ask about other types of substance abuse by using the interviewing technique of symptom expectation:

> *Aside from drinking, what sorts of recreational drugs do you use regularly? Cocaine? Marijuana? Speed? Heroin?*

The phrasing here not only communicates the assumption that your patient has used these drugs but that he uses them on a regular basis; this is an example of symptom exaggeration. The result is that the patient who abuses these drugs occasionally will feel less ashamed to admit such use (e.g., "I don't use them all the time—I've gone on a few coke binges, and I've shot dope a few times, but I keep it under control").

Probing Questions

DSM-5 Criteria for Alcohol Use Disorder

The following list refers to the mnemonic: Tempted With Cognac. For the diagnosis of alcohol use disorder, the patient must meet at least **two** of the following eleven criteria:

- **T**olerance, that is, a need for increasing amounts of alcohol to achieve intoxication
- **W**ithdrawal syndrome
- Loss of **C**ontrol of alcohol use (nine criteria follow):
  - More alcohol ingested than the patient intended
  - Unsuccessful attempts to cut down
  - Much time spent in activities related to obtaining or recovering from the effects of alcohol

- Craving alcohol
- Alcohol use continued despite the patient's knowledge of significant physical or psychological problems caused by its use
- Important social, occupational, or recreational activities given up or reduced because of alcohol use
- Failure to fulfill major role obligations at work, school, or home
- Persistent social and interpersonal problems caused by alcohol
- Recurrent alcohol use in situations in which it is physically hazardous

Once your screening questions have established that your patient has a substance use problem, your next step is to use probing questions to definitively establish the *DSM-5* substance use disorder diagnosis and to assess severity. One way to approach establishing the diagnosis would be to go down the list of criteria, beginning with tolerance, and to simply ask about each one. While this may be time efficient, it tends to produce unreliable information, particularly in the patient who is ashamed of her addiction or is trying to hide the extent of it for other reasons.

The better approach is to ask open-ended questions about your patient's drinking history and transition to specific questions about *DSM-5* criteria as you go along.

Do you remember your first drink?

Alcoholics often remember their first drink vividly and get a twinkle in their eye. For some, this was the first time they ever felt at peace with themselves.

When did you start drinking frequently?

 KEY POINT

The earlier alcoholism began the more severe and refractory the problem is likely to have become. Research shows that 25% of male drinkers have an early-onset form of alcoholism called *type II* alcoholism. This is usually inherited from the father and is a particularly severe form of the disorder, with a high prevalence of violence and comorbid depression and suicidality (Cloninger et al. 1996).

When were you drinking most heavily?

This question allows you to ascertain the sorts of life situations that have been most associated with heavy drinking, and it also serves as a good jumping-off point for a series of questions relating to tolerance, withdrawal, and adverse consequences.

> *Have you found that you've needed more drinks to get the same high?*

Frequent drinkers develop tolerance to the effects of alcohol. A general rule of thumb is that a nonalcoholic person will feel drunk after consuming three to four average drinks on an empty stomach over the course of an hour (Clark 1981). An alcoholic may require two or three times that amount.

> *When you've cut down or stopped drinking for a few days, have you developed problems such as insomnia, the shakes, or convulsions?*

You should become familiar with the usual time course and the symptoms of alcohol withdrawal. Patients generally repeat patterns of withdrawal that they have experienced in the past. This is important for you to know so that you can decide whether to recommend inpatient detoxification to a patient who just stopped drinking.

> *Have you found over the years that you've had trouble controlling your intake of alcohol?*

This is essentially a rephrasing of the "cut-down" question of the CAGE, and it gets at the crucial issue of lack of control of alcohol intake, as expressed in criteria 3 and 4 of the DSM-5.

The next few questions are directed toward finding out whether alcohol use has had a negative effect on the patient's life in some objective way. I stress objective because many alcoholics will deny that they have a subjective problem; via skillful interviewing, you can demonstrate that alcohol has caused problems. In this way, your assessment can, in itself, contribute toward the earliest stage of alcoholism treatment, in which the alcoholic accepts that he has a problem.

In an insightful and cooperative patient, you can get reliable information about adverse effects by asking straightforward questions:

How has your alcoholism affected your relationships?
Your work? Other aspects of your life? Have you gotten
into fights or been arrested because of your drinking?

TIP

When interviewing a patient in denial, however, you will have
to obtain this information indirectly, via the social history and
medical history. A severe alcoholic's social history will be
replete with failed relationships, job changes, and legal difficulties, and his medical history will be significant for emergency room visits or hospitalizations for alcohol-related
injuries. As you glean such information, gingerly introduce
the issue of alcohol use:

You must have felt pretty down when your wife left you.
Was drinking any solace for you then?

Note that this is a normalizing question, with the implicit
message: "Anyone in a similar situation might have reached
for the bottle; that's not something to be ashamed of." If your
patient admits to drinking, follow up with:

Was your drinking an issue with wife? Did she leave
you because of it?

You can use the same technique with other aspects of
the social history. When you hear some clue of alcoholism-
related adverse consequences, ask if alcohol was involved.

Finally, once you've finished getting the remote alcoholism
history, you should ask about recent use. This will help you to
determine the need for detoxification hospitalization and the
extent to which recent alcohol use may be affecting the patient's
mental status. For these questions, you should try to ascertain
quantity of both the amount consumed and the frequency.

> *I need to know about how much you've been drinking*
> *over the past 2 weeks so that I can come up with some*
> *good treatment ideas for you. How many fifths have*
> *you been able to put away per day—one? two? more?*

This question combines a number of defusing strategies.
First, you introduce the question by saying why you're asking

it, not to condemn the patient, but to help him. Second, you appeal to his narcissism by saying "How many fifths have you *been able* to put away?" Finally, you use symptom exaggeration by suggesting a degree of use higher than you expect: one, two, or more fifths per day.

"BLAME IT ON THE ALCOHOL" TECHNIQUE

Another good way of helping your patient ponder ways in which alcohol might have become a real problem (described by White and Epston 1990) is to give it an exterior identity, almost as if it were a separate person. This way, you and your patient can join forces against an outside "enemy." For example, you can ask such questions as "If it were possible, would you like to limit the way that alcohol pushes you around? ... How has alcohol been tricking you into withdrawing and avoiding people? ... What would life be like if alcohol weren't around anymore?"

SPECIAL TECHNIQUES IN DUAL DIAGNOSIS

If your patient has a substance abuse problem, chances are high that he has another psychiatric disorder, as well. According to the largest American epidemiologic study to look at this question, 37% of alcoholics and 53% of drug abusers have had another psychiatric disorder at some point in their lives (Regier et al. 1990). Using a particularly common example, that of depression combined with alcoholism, two disorders can interact with each other in two ways: Depression can drive a person to drink, or drinking can cause depression, either directly via a depressant effect on the nerve cells or indirectly via the psychosocial chaos that alcoholism causes.

Patients with dual diagnoses are complicated, and you may need to schedule two sessions to complete your diagnostic assessment. Here are some suggestions for making these assessments easier. For ease of presentation, I use the example of depression and alcoholism, but any other dual diagnoses can be approached similarly.

When was your longest period of sobriety?

You want to identify a period of sobriety lasting at least 2 months, preferably longer. Refer to that period in further questions.

How was your life going during that period? Were you suffering from depression or anxiety?

Try to determine if the patient met DSM-5 criteria for a major depressive episode during her sobriety. It doesn't count if she was depressed for only a few weeks after she stopped drinking and the depression resolved on its own. That's the typical course of alcohol-induced depression. Look for depression that was separated from their alcohol use by at least 1 month.

Why did you begin drinking again?
Was it because of depression, or just because the temptation to drink was too great?
Which do you think is a bigger problem for you, alcohol dependence or depression?

Sometimes, the patient will have a good sense as to which disorder is his central problem. However, you should be wary of the antisocial patient who tries to convince you that he is depressed (rather than alcoholic) to obtain disability benefits or a psychiatric admission.

Assessing Psychotic Disorders

A body seriously out of equilibrium, either with itself or with its environment, perishes outright. Not so a mind. Madness and suffering can set themselves no limit.

George Santayana

The first important point for novice interviewers is that psychosis and schizophrenia are not interchangeable. *Psychosis* is a general term referring to disordered processing of thought and impaired grasp of reality. As such, psychosis can occur as a part of many psychiatric syndromes other than schizophrenia, including:

- Depression
- Mania
- Overwhelming stress *(brief reactive psychosis)*
- Dissociative disorders
- Dementia and delirium
- Substance intoxication or withdrawal
- Personality disorders (PDs)

In terms of the rapid diagnostic evaluation, this means that you must ask every patient you interview, not only those whom you suspect of having schizophrenia, screening questions about psychotic ideation.

The second useful point, related to the first, is that there are two types of psychotic patients: (a) those who are obviously psychotic and (b) those whose psychoses are not obvious. In most outpatient settings, the typical patient will not appear psychotic at first glance. He will speak coherently, will not volunteer any delusional material, and will not appear to be hallucinating. However, many of these patients will have a subtle or hidden psychosis that will require a number of screening questions to uncover. These screening questions and techniques are described in the first part of this chapter.

On the other hand, patients who *are* obviously psychotic don't require subtle screening questions. Instead, you will ask probing questions to better understand the precise type of psychosis with which you are dealing. In the second part of this chapter, I define the more common thought disorders and then describe strategies for ascertaining which are present in a particular patient.

GENERAL SCREENING QUESTIONS

When you are interviewing a patient who speaks coherently and has a good grasp of reality, it is tempting to skip questions regarding psychosis. This is a mistake, because hidden psychosis is common, especially in major depression, dementia, and substance abuse. In addition, a nonpsychotic patient may have a history of psychosis, which in turn may influence your diagnosis or treatment.

Two good initial questions are as follows:

> *Have you had any experiences like dreaming when you're awake?*
> *Have you had any strange or odd experiences lately that you can't explain?*

Patients who answer "no" to both of these questions may still be psychotic, and if you suspect this, you should follow up with

> *Do you ever hear or see things that other people can't hear or see?*

This asks directly about auditory and visual hallucinations but is more graceful than the old standby, "Do you hear voices?"

TIP

Not all people who hear voices have a psychiatric syndrome. Epidemiological research has documented that 3% to 4% of people in the general population report a history of auditory hallucinations (AHs), and less than one half of them meet criteria for schizophrenia or dissociative disorder. In one study comparing patient with nonpatient "voice hearers," the nonpatients often reported the onset of AHs before age 12, and 93% of them thought that the voices were predominantly positive (Honig et al. 1998).

Have people been harassing you or trying to harm you?

This question screens for paranoid ideation in a nonjudgmental way. You are not asking your patient if she is paranoid, but rather whether she feels others are wronging her. A subtly paranoid patient may welcome this chance to vent her complaints about the Federal Bureau of Investigation's (FBI's) wiretapping activities.

Does it seem that strangers look at you a lot or make comments about you?

This is a screen for ideas of reference, a common psychotic delusion in which the patient believes that apparently neutral events have a special significance or communication for her. Ideas of reference can be very subtle and difficult to diagnose, as the following vignette illustrates.

CLINICAL VIGNETTE

An intern was admitting a 63-year-old widowed woman with major depression. The patient had become increasingly depressed since her husband died 1 year earlier, and she had not responded to antidepressants thus far, prompting an admission for more intensive diagnostic evaluation and treatment. After establishing criteria for major depression, the intern asked her screening questions for psychotic ideation:

Interviewer: Do you ever feel that people you don't know are looking at you or making comments about you?

Patient: No.
Interviewer: Do you ever hear voices or see things that other people can't see?
Patient: No.
Interviewer: Has anyone been bothering you or harassing you?
Patient: Just the kids in the neighborhood.
Interviewer: What have they been doing?
Patient: What kids do, yelling and carrying on.

At this point, the intern was tempted to drop this topic and move on to another section of the interview, but she had a vague sense that there was something more to this story than the "carrying on" of neighborhood kids.

Interviewer: What sorts of things have the kids been yelling?
Patient: Saying bad things about me.
Interviewer: What sorts of things?
Patient: Oh, that I'm a prostitute. That I run a whorehouse. They're yelling it day and night.

As it turned out, the patient had major depression with psychotic features (AHs and ideas of reference) and required combination therapy with an antidepressant and a neuroleptic before she improved.

TIP

You can also make any of these questions sound less threatening by using smooth transitions and normalization techniques, covered in Chapters 4 and 6.

For example, your patient has just told you how depressed she has been, and you follow up:

Deep depression sometimes causes people to have strange experiences, such as hearing voices or feeling that others are trying to harm them. Has that happened to you?

Of course, you can use many other symptoms as springboards for asking about psychosis, including the following:

• Anxiety: Has your anxiety gotten to the point where your imagination is working in overdrive, so that you hear voices or think people are trying to harm you?

- Substance abuse: Have these drugs ever caused your mind to play tricks on you, such as…?
- Dementia: When you misplace things around the house, do you ever suspect that someone's been stealing them?

PROBING QUESTIONS: HOW TO DIAGNOSE SCHIZOPHRENIA

There is both good news and bad news about diagnosing schizophrenia. The good news is that it is fairly easy; the bad news is that we have made it seem complicated by creating a plethora of colorful, though confusing, terms for describing psychosis. To illustrate, here is a partial list of terms in current use:

- Tangentiality
- Circumstantiality
- Distractibility
- Derailment
- Looseness of associations (LOAs)
- Disjointed speech
- Flight of ideas
- Pressure of speech
- Racing thoughts
- Word salad
- Incoherence
- Loss of goal
- Illogical thinking
- Rambling
- Thought blocking
- Poverty of speech
- Poverty of thought
- Poverty of content
- Nonsequiturs
- Perseveration
- Clanging
- Neologism
- Paraphasias
- Echolalia
- Stilted speech
- Self-reference
- Persecutory (paranoid) delusions
- Delusion of jealousy

- Erotomania
- Delusion of control
- Delusion of guilt or sin
- Delusion of grandiosity
- Delusion of mind reading
- Ideas of reference
- Delusion of replacement
- Nihilistic delusion
- Somatic delusion
- Thought broadcasting
- Thought insertion
- Thought withdrawal
- Magical thinking
- Poor reality testing
- Attending to internal stimuli

   To begin to simplify this semantic onslaught, it's helpful to review the basic criteria for schizophrenia.

SCHIZOPHRENIA

The *DSM-5* criteria for schizophrenia are listed in Table 27.1.

Delusions (Disorders of Thought Content)

A common and useful distinction is made between TC and TP. Both TC and TP can be impaired in psychosis. Impaired TP is covered under the speech disorganization criterion for

TABLE 27.1. *DSM-5* Criteria for Schizophrenia

Requires two symptoms for 1 mo, plus 5 mo of prodromal or residual symptoms. At least one symptom must be one of the three highlighted core symptoms (delusions, hallucinations, speech disorganization)

Mnemonic: **D**elusions **H**erald **S**chizophrenic's **B**ad **N**ews

Delusions

Hallucinations

Speech/thought disorganization

Behavior disorganization

Negative symptoms

Data from American Psychiatric Association. (2013). *Diagnostic and Statistical Manual of Mental Disorders*, 5th ed. Washington, DC: American Psychiatric Association.

schizophrenia later in this chapter. *Impaired TC* refers to delusional thinking. A *delusion* is a belief about the world that most people would agree is impossible. Most delusions fit into two broad categories: paranoid delusions and grandiose delusions.

Paranoid Delusions

According to a World Health Organization study of 811 individuals with schizophrenia worldwide (McKenna 1994), paranoia was the most common single delusion, affecting 60% of patients. Paranoid patients believe that people are harassing them, chasing them, spying on them, spreading rumors about them, or trying to kill them. Large organizations are frequently thought to be involved, such as the FBI, the Central Intelligence Agency, or the Mafia. For example, a young man believed that his wife was an undercover FBI agent determined to kill him for having "blown her cover."

A number of subcategories of paranoid delusions may or may not be present in a particular psychotic patient.

DELUSIONS (OR IDEAS) OF REFERENCE

The patient having delusions of reference believes that casual events have a special (and usually dangerous) significance in reference to her. Thus, strangers waiting at a subway stop may be thought to be staring at or talking about her. In its more severe form, the patient may believe that people on the radio or TV are discussing him or speaking directly to him.

NOTE

Delusions of reference can also occur as a feature of grandiose delusions but are most common in paranoia. For example, a woman thought she was being pursued by a hit squad. At work, she noted that coworkers appeared to be whispering things about the plot against her. While she was driving, she perceived an elaborate system of communication among other cars, in which turn signals and headlights were used to indicate her precise location to the killers.

Following are questions for delusions of reference:

> *Have you noticed that strangers on the street have been looking at you or talking about you?*
> *Have you felt that people on the radio or TV were talking about you in their reports, or giving you special messages?*
> *Do you get any messages from books or newspapers?*

Delusions of Control or Influence

The patient with delusions of control believes he is being controlled by some outside force. For example, an immigrant from Latin America believed he was being forced to stay in the United States by the President, who he believed was transmitting ensnaring rays through his television set.

Delusions of Replacement (Capgras Syndrome)

A delusion of replacement is a belief that important people in one's life have been replaced by impostors. For example, a woman believed that her mother had been replaced by a stranger who was in league with a fringe religious group attempting to seize possession of her home.

Delusions of Jealousy

A delusion of jealousy is a belief that one's spouse is unfaithful, despite no supporting evidence.

Somatic Delusions

The patient having somatic delusions believes that she has an illness or is being poisoned despite the absence of medical evidence. If you suspect somatic delusions, you can elicit them with these questions:

> *Are you worried about your body?*
> *Do you think you have cancer or another serious disease?*
> *Do you suspect that someone has poisoned you?*
> *Has anyone been altering your medication?*
> *Is a particular person responsible for your physical symptoms?*

NOTE

Many of these questions are also appropriate for assessing somatization disorder, which is not a psychotic disorder.

Somatic delusions frequently occur as an associated feature of depression.

CLINICAL VIGNETTE

A 38-year-old married woman presented to the emergency room with symptoms of anxiety and depression. In the interview, she said she was afraid that she had HIV infection and syphilis, despite several recent normal blood test results. These fears began after an extramarital affair in which her partner had not used a condom. The patient began to ruminate about the possibility that she had contracted a venereal disease. She became convinced that her entire neighborhood knew about it and that, because of this, she had brought "doom" on her family. These fears led her to consider overdosing on medication as a suicide attempt.

Grandiose Delusions

Often seen during a manic episode, grandiose delusions entail the belief that one has special powers and is accomplishing (or will accomplish) extraordinary things. Two common types of grandiosity exist: religious and technological.

Religious Delusions

A religious delusion is a very common type of grandiose delusion in which the patient believes she is God-like. In an example of this, a 40-year-old woman was evaluated in the emergency room after having been found standing in the middle of traffic holding her hands high above her head, palms facing oncoming cars. She explained this behavior by saying she was the Messiah and was healing all the people in their cars during rush hour.

The following questions are for religious delusions:

Do you consider yourself to be a religious person?
Do you have a special relationship with God?
Do you have any special religious powers or abilities?

Technological Delusions

The patient with technological delusions believes that he is somehow connected to computers or other electrical appliances, allowing him to exert immense power. For example, a 30-year-old former taxi driver described a business idea. He proposed to coordinate large fleets of taxis that would be in business with restaurants, theaters, and workplaces in a large city. Because all of these settings had financial stakes in people's arriving and leaving, they would be happy to pay the patient for his services. "I wouldn't need any staff," he continued. "I could do it all myself, through the license plates." His intention was to have a transmitter inserted into his brain that could send messages to each cabbie via receivers in the license plates. In an effort to reality test, it was pointed out to him that no such device existed. He responded, "I have it already," pointing to what looked like a large pimple on his forehead.

General Interviewing Tips for Asking About Delusions

Nonjudgmental Questions

The general strategy in interviewing patients you suspect to be paranoid is to portray yourself as nonjudgmental. If you come across as critical, you are likely to become part of their delusional system.

Has anyone treated you badly or annoyed you in any way that was unusual?
Has anyone been paying particular attention to you, watching you, or talking about you?

Both of these questions imply that you want to become the patient's ally, rather than his enemy.

Counterprojective Statements

In some cases, your patient may be so paranoid that he clearly distrusts you, incorporating you into his delusional system. A counterprojective statement can work well here. In it, you explicitly acknowledge and sympathize with your patient's projection (Havens 1986; see also Chapter 3).

CLINICAL VIGNETTE

Interviewer: What brought you into the hospital?
Patient: (Looking suspicious) You would know, wouldn't you?
Interviewer: I don't know. That's why I'm asking.
Patient: I was forced here for surveillance. The Secret Service is involved. That's all I'm saying, because I know my rights.
Interviewer: (Using counterprojective statement) And then here I come, looking all official in my coat and tie, saying I'm a psychiatrist. ... You probably think I'm part of the Secret Service too, which would be understandable.
Patient: Can anyone hear us?
Interviewer: Nope. The door's closed.
Patient: Okay, here's what happened. (Patient opens up significantly.)

Techniques for Reality Testing

Reality testing refers to your efforts to see how strongly your patient believes in his delusion. It helps you to determine the severity of a psychotic disorder and also will help you monitor the patient's response to treatment. Studies of the natural course of delusions have revealed three phases (Sacks et al. 1974):

1. An initial phase in which the patient is totally convinced of the belief
2. An intermediate, "double-awareness" phase in which the patient begins to question the delusion
3. A nondelusional phase

Sensitive questioning will help you determine just which phase your patient is in. Rather than labeling her belief as delusional, frame the delusion in such a way that it is normalized.

> TIP

Frame delusions in terms of the patient's *imagination:*
  Do you think your imagination has been getting the best of you?
  Has your imagination been working in overdrive?
  Have you been imagining things?
Blame it on the *mind:*
  Has your mind been playing tricks on you lately?
  Do you think your mind pulled a fast one on you when you thought that?
Ask about *fantasy:*
  Do you think you might have been fantasizing any of this?

Hallucinations

Hallucinations occur in approximately one half of all patients with schizophrenia (Flaum 1995), but they also commonly occur in depression, bipolar disorder, substance abuse disorders, dissociative disorders, and dementia.

> *Have you had any unusual experiences lately, such as hearing voices when there's no one else around?*

Once you've established the presence of AHs, ask in more detail about the quality and content of the voices. Adopting an interested and curious attitude often helps break the patient's guard.

> *I've never heard voices before, and I'm curious what it's like for you. Tell me more about these voices. Is there one voice or more than one? Is it male or female? If I were to put a microphone to the voices, what exactly would I hear?*

Ask specifically if the patient is hearing command hallucinations.

> *Are the voices telling you to do anything?*
> *Are they saying bad things about you, or telling you to hurt yourself or anyone else?*

Another way to ask about hallucinations is to ask in the context of your questions about depression.

Sometimes when people get very depressed, their mind plays tricks on them, and they think they hear things that others can't hear. Has that happened to you?

This diminishes the embarrassing nature of a positive response by normalizing the experience (see Chapter 4).

Have you heard, seen, smelled, or felt things that other people couldn't?

Here, you are asking about all the major types of hallucinations in one fell swoop: auditory, visual, olfactory, and tactile.

Disorganized Speech

What the *DSM-5* terms *disorganized speech* is also known as *disorder of thought process* or *formal thought disorder,* because there is a disorder of the form, rather than the content, of thought.

To understand how to recognize a disorder of TP, consider your own thinking style. When you think or talk about something, you do so in a linear and logical way—that is, one thought leads naturally to another. In addition, you normally think your thoughts at a comfortable speed, so that when you are speaking, other people can understand you. Patients with a formal thought disorder do not make sense, because their thinking is neither linear nor logical, and there is often a disorder in the speed of their thoughts.

All of the jargon concerning disorganized speech can be fit into one of two clusters: the LOA cluster and the velocity cluster.

Looseness of Association Cluster

LOA refers to a veering off from the subject at hand. There is a range of severity of LOA, from circumstantiality at one end to word salad at the other. A patient who exhibits any one of these qualities to a significant degree fulfills the disorganized speech criteria for schizophrenia.

Although a number of terms describe different degrees of LOA, the most useful thing to do clinically is to document that the patient exhibits LOA; describe it as mild, moderate, or severe; and give a brief example (verbatim from the interview) in the write-up. This allows you to track the patient's response to treatment and enables other clinicians who read your notes to compare their observations with yours.

Circumstantiality

The patient with a circumstantial thinking style makes many digressions in her speech and adds extraneous details. These digressions are usually related, however distantly, to the subject matter at hand, and after a while, the speaker will return to that subject matter. You'll recognize a circumstantial style because you will feel impatient and will be forced to interrupt often and redirect to finish the interview within a reasonable period.

Circumstantiality is not necessarily pathologic. Nonpatients who are circumstantial are popularly termed *long winded*. College lecturers and great storytellers are famous for circumstantiality. Within the realm of the *DSM-5*, demented or anxious patients often present with circumstantial style.

Tangentiality

Whereas circumstantial speech is basically understandable, though tedious, tangential speech begins to approach incoherence. Digressions are more abrupt and less obviously relevant to the subject at hand. Unlike the circumstantial patient, the tangential patient will never return to the topic of your question, no matter how long you wait. This usually indicates either psychosis or dementia.

Example

> **Interviewer:** *Have you ever been hospitalized before?*
> **Patient:** *I went into the hospital in 1992 and again in 1993. I'm a wanderer, and where people tell me to go, there I will go. Last night, I wandered into the room at the end of the hall here and there were some flies buzzing around. I told the nurse about it but she didn't see that as her job, so I swatted them. Do you have any control over the hygienic circumstances here?*

Here, the patient has veered from the subject of her PPH to that of flies in the unit. However, she is basically coherent and with frequent redirection will be able to give meaningful historical information.

Related Term

Rambling: The same as tangentiality, but it is classically reserved for describing demented patients.

Looseness of Association

LOA is a more severe version of tangentiality. The patient makes statements that lead to other statements in a very loose way, so that the associative leaps are unclear. There are clearly associations going on somewhere in your patient's mind, but you can't make them out.

Example

> *Interviewer: What brings you into the clinic today?*
> *Patient: I don't know. I might be thrown out. Benito Mussolini actually came alive out in the waiting room. I figured it out. There was a picture in a book. If it's not my mother, it could have been Hitler. What if that was one of his armed guards. Mussolini was hanging from a tree! Thank you for letting me reason it out. Oh, that's another thing that I wanted to talk to you about... being brainwashed. I didn't buy the Beatles tape, I never did.*

The patient is following some pretty disjointed associations in his brain, and it is unlikely that you will be able to obtain a meaningful history. However, the sentences are grammatically correct and internally coherent.

Related Terms

> *Derailment: Equivalent term.*
> *Disjointed speech: Equivalent term.*
> *Loss of goal: Refers to speech that doesn't lead to any particular point and that doesn't come close to answering your question; the cause is generally LOA.*
> *Flight of ideas: Refers to LOA when thoughts are moving rapidly.*
> *Racing thoughts: Refers to coherent thoughts that are moving rapidly.*

Word Salad

Word salad is an extreme version of LOA, in which the changes in topic are so extreme and the associations so loose that the resulting speech is completely incoherent. It differs from LOA in that the digressions occur within a particular sentence, between words, in addition to between sentences.

Example

> *Interviewer: How did you end up at the hospital?*
> *Patient: It was a section 8 day. I'm not saying there's a utilitarian. I just had no patience with the curfew system.*
> *Interviewer: Why did you go to the halfway house?*
> *Patient: I'm helpless as a savant idiot. There was a circulation of their publicity. Would you like it?*
> *Interviewer: What kind of work did you do?*
> *Patient: I worked in computer electricities. It was a nondilated baccalaureate. I mean a nondiluted baccalaureate.*

In this case, individual sentences make no sense. You feel almost as though your patient is speaking a different language.

Related Terms

> *Incoherence: The direct consequence of word salad.*
> *Non sequiturs: Out-of-context words placed into sentences.*
> *Neologisms: Spontaneously made up words that often accompany word salad; "nondiluted baccalaureate" is an example.*
> *Clang associations: Associations based on the sounds of words.*

Velocity Cluster

In addition to an impaired ability to associate one thought with another, psychotic patients often show an abnormality in the speed or rate of production of their thoughts. This ranges from *mutism* at one end of the continuum to *flight of ideas* at the other.

Mutism

A patient exhibiting *mutism* simply will not speak. This may mean that he is having few, if any, thoughts, which can occur as a negative symptom of schizophrenia. It can occur in the catatonia of affective disorders. Mutism may also be a response to a delusional system.

Example

A young woman who was admitted to a psychiatric unit remained mute for several days until she began responding to antipsychotic medication. She later related that she had been told by God that her absolute silence was the only thing preventing the collision of matter with antimatter and the consequent annihilation of the world.

Poverty of Thought

Your patient has *poverty of thought* if he offers very little spontaneous speech and if his answers to questions are with the minimum number of words required. You have to distinguish this type of psychotic patient from the angry and resistant patient who is admitted involuntarily to a hospital unit or who is under court order to seek therapy. The psychotic patient will often show other negative symptoms of schizophrenia, such as poor hygiene, flat affect, or a history of social isolation.

Example (from Andreasen 1979)

Interviewer: Were you working at all before you came to the hospital?
Patient: No.
Interviewer: What kinds of jobs have you had in the past?
Patient: Oh, some janitor jobs, painting.
Interviewer: What kind of work do you do?
Patient: I don't. I don't do any kind of work. That's silly.
Interviewer: How far did you go in school?
Patient: I'm still in eleventh grade.
Interviewer: How old are you?
Patient: Eighteen.

Related Terms

Poverty of speech: Equivalent term.
Lack of spontaneous speech: Equivalent term.
Thought blocking: Your patient begins to say something, then stops in midthought and forgets what he was going to say.

Interviewing Strategies

You will recognize poverty of thought easily. You will find yourself asking questions far more frequently than usual, because the patient provides no information beyond a minimal response to each question. It is often difficult in these patients to discover whether there are any positive symptoms of schizophrenia, such as delusions or hallucinations. One way to elicit a flow of spontaneous speech is to ask open-ended and provocative questions about general topics:

> *What do you think about the legalization of marijuana?*
> *Who was your favorite teacher in high school?*
> *What kind of person are you?*
> *Do you believe in God?*

Poverty of Content

Your patient may produce a copious amount of speech but somehow communicate very little information or discernible meaning. This is usually because the speech is overly abstract.

Interviewer: *Why do you think it would be better for you to move out of your mother's house?*

Patient: *It would be exactly because of the things we were talking about before, and which I was talking to some of the other counselors about. I think we were talking about supervised housing and that would be related to how I might find another place to live, away from my mother, and that would change who I would communicate with. Of course my mother is a person and she would like to communicate with me, and I communicate with her all the time. I think the difference is that it would be a different situation and in a different place. I would have to talk to my case worker about moving. I'm sure my mother wants it, too.*

You find yourself scratching your head. Your question hasn't been answered, but not because the patient has veered away from the topic of moving, as in LOA. His response has remained on topic, but he hasn't said anything meaningful about it.

Related Term

Perseveration: Your patient talks but dwells on a single idea or preoccupation over and over. This can be seen in both OCD and dementia, as well as in psychosis.

Racing Thoughts

Racing thoughts refers to the subjective sense of one's thoughts going so fast that they're hard to keep track of, which may or may not be associated with pressured speech. Some patients who are not talkative report having racing thoughts, often occurring with anxiety. Racing thoughts also occur commonly in substance-abusing patients undergoing detoxification. To ascertain the presence of racing thoughts, ask:

> *Are you having trouble keeping up with your thoughts?*
> *Are your thoughts moving so quickly that you can't keep up with them?*

Related Term

Pressured speech: This is very rapid speech that is difficult to interrupt and is often loud and intense. When racing thoughts are converted directly into speech, the result is pressured speech, and the diagnosis is almost always mania.

Example

> *Interviewer:* How did you come into the hospital?
> *Patient:* (While pacing back and forth in her room) I could remember taking care of business. I felt like I was here, there, and everywhere. I know I was not sick, because a sick human cannot remember everything there is to remember, like that (she snaps her fingers), and I could, and do you know why? Ask the Master, the Master is everywhere, the Master knows everything, the Master is God, and that's why I'm still here. ...

Flight of Ideas

Flight of ideas is a special case of LOA when the incoherent associations occur very rapidly. As such, it is not necessarily equivalent to either *pressured speech,* which can refer to quite coherent but rapid speech, or *racing thoughts,* which can also be coherent.

Disorder of Behavior (Disorganized Behavior)

Disorganized behavior is diagnosed primarily by observation during the interview, although obtaining information from outside sources is often helpful. Observational clues include poor grooming, body odor, and bizarre clothing combinations. Another clue can be obtained by asking your patient to complete a simple task. This can be done in the context of the cognitive examination (see Chapter 21) or simply by asking your patient for his insurance or appointment card. A typically disorganized patient will pull out a torn, bulging purse or wallet and will rummage through a seemingly random array of material before finding anything.

Paucity of Thought, Affect, and Behavior (Negative Symptoms)

Symptoms of schizophrenia have been classically divided into *positive* symptoms (e.g., delusions, hallucinations) and *negative* symptoms (e.g., flat affect, apathy, asociality, poverty of speech) (Andreasen 1982). The patient with negative symptoms will tend to say very little, speak slowly, show very little affect, have few spontaneous movements, and be poorly groomed. His social history will reflect lack of motivation and inability to persist in school or work activities. Family members may report that he spends most of his time sitting around, doing little, and that he has few, if any, friends.

28 ▼ Assessing Neurocognitive Disorders (Dementia and Delirium)

Screening Questions

- Orientation
  What's your full name?
  Where are we right now?
  What's today's date?
- Short-term memory

  Repeat these three words: ball, chair, purple. Keep them in mind, because I'm going to ask you to repeat them in a couple of minutes.

- Personal and general information
  Name the last three presidents.
  Who was George Washington? Abraham Lincoln? Martin Luther King, Jr.? Shakespeare?
  When was World War II? When was John F. Kennedy assassinated?
  What's your address and phone number?
  What are your spouse's/children's/siblings'/ parents' names and birthdays?
  When and where were you married?

One of the major terminology changes of DSM-5 was to classify dementia and delirium as "neurocognitive disorders." Delirium is still called delirium, but dementia has now become "major neurocognitive disorder," while a milder form of dementia has been called "mild neurocognitive disorder."

In Chapter 21, I outline a rapid cognitive examination with components based on studies showing them to be effective in identifying patients with cognitive deficits. In this chapter, I show you how to tailor your questions to the patient who may have either delirium or dementia. In *delirium*, attention is impaired, and all of the cognitive processes are therefore also impaired. In *dementia*, attention is intact, but the cognitive processes, particularly memory, are impaired.

With this in mind, let's look at the *DSM-5* criteria for both dementia and delirium and then review interview techniques for making the diagnoses.

DELIRIUM

Impaired Attention

The key to diagnosing delirium is establishing an impairment in your patient's attention. A delirious patient has difficulty sustaining his attention for a significant period. As in Chapter 21, I discourage reliance on traditional and unproved tests of attention, such as the subtraction of serial sevens test (SSST), and instead encourage you to rely on your patient's ability to respond to routine questions (Table 28.1).

Most of your interviews with delirious patients will occur in a hospital setting, often when you have been asked to see the patient by the primary care physician. In such settings, there are two types of delirious patients: the loud and the quiet. The loud delirious patient will typically be rambling incoherently and may be struggling against restraints in an effort to leave the hospital bed or to pull out intravenous lines.

The quiet delirious patient, on the other hand, requires some verbal probing to make a diagnosis. It's often helpful to

TABLE 28.1. *DSM-5* Criteria for Delirium

(Note: The *DSM-5* specifies a number of different types of delirium, but the core diagnostic criteria as listed below do not change.)

Disturbance of awareness (i.e., reduced clarity of awareness of the environment) with reduced ability to focus, sustain, or shift attention

A change in cognition (e.g., memory deficit, disorientation, language disturbance) or the development of a perceptual disturbance that is not better accounted for by a preexisting dementia

A disturbance developing over a short period (usually hours to days) and fluctuating during the course of the day

There is a medical cause

Mnemonic: **Medical FRAT**

> **Medical** cause
> **F**luctuating course
> **R**ecent onset
> **A**ttentional impairment
> **T**hinking impairment

Adapted from American Psychiatric Association. (2013). *Diagnostic and Statistical Manual of Mental Disorders*, 5th ed. Washington, DC: American Psychiatric Association.

begin by saying nothing—that is, by walking into the room and observing your patient's behavior. A person with normal cognitive abilities will generally look at you and make some kind of greeting and then wait for you to respond. A delirious patient may glance at you briefly and then pay little attention to you. He may be talking softly to himself. He may be looking all around the room, tracking a hallucinated bird or insect.

Hello, Mr. Brown. What brings you into the hospital?

The patient should be able to answer coherently. If the patient answers incoherently, you have to assess the nature of the incoherence. In many mental disorders, the patient's attention is normal, but the TP or TC is disordered in some way.

Of the following three clinical vignettes, for example, only the third describes true delirium.

CLINICAL VIGNETTE 1

A hospitalized psychotic patient gave me this answer:

> *I got tricked into this, but I won't complain, because exactly at this moment, there are stereoscopic beams coming into this room from transmitters, and they are focused on my brain cells. Please stay still, because the beams are coming around you now.*

On further questioning, it was apparent that the patient was suffering a fixed, bizarre, paranoid delusion, but his attention was quite intact.

CLINICAL VIGNETTE 2

Another patient responded with the following:

> *This is no hospital, this is my home, because I can see my granddaughter out there. She was just about to bring me in some tea. Oh, I know you. You're that man they sent in to help me.*

The patient had a profound impairment of short-term memory, secondary to Alzheimer's dementia. She could not remember that she was in a hospital, but her attention was intact.

CLINICAL VIGNETTE 3

A truly delirious patient responded:

> *Hello! (He looked up at the ceiling.) Something... what is that? (He was quickly oblivious to my presence. I asked again why he was in the hospital.) I'm in the hospital for... (He looked confused.) There's something here in the hospital, my son said... (He looked at me again as if scrutinizing me, then turned away, again seeming to forget about my presence as he looked at the ceiling.)*

The patient seemed to understand my words, but he had no ability to maintain his attention to me or to continue a single train of thought. As it turned out, the patient was in delirium tremens after having abruptly stopped his prescribed alprazolam (Xanax) 3 days earlier.

Change in Cognition

Almost all delirious patients will have great difficulty with the three-object recall task, as their attention is too impaired to register the words in the first place. Visual or auditory hallucinations are also extremely common.

Recent Onset and Fluctuating Course

You have to rely on gathering history from sources other than the patient to ascertain that the onset of the cognitive impairment has been relatively recent (days to weeks), excluding the diagnosis of dementia. With regard to fluctuations in attention, the best way for you to determine this is to examine the patient at least twice during the day. If you can't see the patient again, ask other caregivers to report whether she was able to coherently answer simple questions (e.g., "Why are you here?").

NEUROCOGNITIVE DISORDER

Interviewing Family Members

Interviews with family members and other informants are vitally important in making the diagnosis of neurocognitive disorder (NCD) (Table 28.2). This is because the patient himself will often deny or minimize his memory problem and, at any rate, an affected patient's self-reported history will be unreliable. Therefore, the best way to diagnose NCD is by combining the MSE with interviews of informants. In fact, studies that have compared the two approaches (the MSE vs. informant questionnaires) have found informant interviews to be the more sensitive of the two (Harwood et al. 1997).

When you interview family members, you should begin by asking them to compare the patient's current cognitive abilities with the patient's abilities of 10 years ago. This will put the focus on a gradual decline in functioning, which is what differentiates NCD from delirium.

The general form of your questioning should follow the format of the Informant Questionnaire on Cognitive Decline in the Elderly (IQCODE; Jorm 1991), from which most of the following questions are derived. Ask the following questions:

Compared with 10 years ago, how is this person at:

- Remembering things that have happened recently?
- Remembering where things are usually kept?
- Remembering things about family and friends, such as names, occupations, birthdays, or addresses?
- Making decisions on everyday matters?
- Handling financial matters?
- Finding the right word when talking about things?
- Knowing how to do everyday things around the house, such as cooking and cleaning?

TABLE 28.2. *DSM-5* Criteria for Dementia

(Note: The *DSM-5* specifies a number of different types of NCD, but the core diagnostic criteria as listed below do not change.)
Mnemonic:
Memory **LAPSE**
1. **M**emory
2. **L**anguage
3. **A**ttention (complex)
4. **P**erceptual-motor
5. **S**ocial cognition
6. **E**xecutive function
At least one of the six criteria is required.

Adapted from American Psychiatric Association. (2013). *Diagnostic and Statistical Manual of Mental Disorders*, 5th ed. Washington, DC: American Psychiatric Association.

- Following social cues, such as making appropriate comments in conversations? Has there been a personality change?

Interviewing the Patient

In order to diagnose an NCD, *DSM-5* requires you to demonstrate that your patient is significantly impaired in at least one of six "neurocognitive domains." The domains are as follows:

1. Memory
2. Complex attention
3. Executive function
4. Language
5. Perceptual-motor
6. Social cognition

For those of you used to DSM-IV, you'll notice that diagnosing dementia is now more complicated. It used to be that the key piece of the diagnosis was a memory impairment, followed by one of four other impairments. But with DSM-5, memory impairment is no longer a requirement, and you have to assess the six domains, some of which are somewhat confusing.

1. **Memory.** Though DSM-5 may longer require memory loss for the diagnosis, it would be the very rare person with dementia who does not have this impairment. I suggested an approach to assessing memory in Chapter 21, which I won't repeat here. Remember that before you go too far in your examination, do your basic delirium screen (see above). If the patient is delirious, you won't be able to conclude anything about NCD based on the examination; if the patient is awake and attentive, proceed with the rest of the cognitive examination as outlined in Chapter 21.
2. **Complex Attention.** Problems with complex attention are different from the impaired attention that we see in delirium. The patient might be able to sustain attention long enough to have a simple conversation with you (unlike the delirious patient). But put them in a situation with multiple sources of stimuli at the same time, the attentional abilities get stressed. You will have a hard time

establishing this by talking to the patient, but high-yield questions to ask informants include:

Does he tend to get easily distracted from a conversation when other things are going on in the room, like other conversations, or music, or kids playing?
Does she seem to have a harder time focusing on tasks that used to be simple, like repeating a phone number that she just heard, or writing down something while taking on the phone?

3. **Executive function.** Here, you are testing a complex ability—the ability to plan and think abstractly. A deficit in executive functioning will often come through during the history. This is especially true if the patient was employed as the dementia began. You will hear about job difficulties, inefficiencies accomplishing tasks that were once easy, and the like. Occasionally, it may be difficult to distinguish this from the personality changes that occur in dementia—new-onset indifference and irritability can play havoc with job performance, especially in service-oriented jobs.

To test executive functioning, you can use the three-step command (described earlier). However, the classic screening test for this is the clock-drawing task, in which you give the patient a sheet of paper with a circle and a dot in the center and tell her

I'd like you to write in all the numbers of a clock and then to draw in the hands to represent 2:30.

Patients with poor executive function may exhibit a number of different errors, such as bunching numbers too closely together, skipping or repeating numbers, or drawing the hands incorrectly. One potential problem with this task is that performance varies by education (Ainslie 1993). Thus, you should give it only to patients with at least some high school education. Otherwise, you may falsely interpret a poor clock as meaning that a patient is cognitively impaired, when in fact he is merely poorly educated.

4. **Language problems** (also known as aphasia). The most common language problem in dementia is a difficulty finding the right word for something. If present, word-finding difficulty will have become apparent over the

course of the interview. In mild cases, the right word seems to be on the tip of the patient's tongue:

> **Interviewer:** *Who was George Washington?*
> **Patient:** *Oh, he was that man, the uh… top man of the whole thing.*
> **Interviewer:** *What do you mean by the "top man"?*
> **Patient:** *The whole country voted for him.*
> **Interviewer:** *Do you mean the "president"?*
> **Patient:** *Right! The president!*

A specific screening test for aphasia is to point out common objects in the room and ask your patient to name them (e.g., your pen, your watch, or a chair). However, doing so will only pick up severe cases of aphasia. Interviewing informants is often an excellent way to pick up an early aphasia.

5. **Perceptual-motor problems** (often termed apraxia). This refers to difficulty accomplishing simple, everyday activities despite an intact nervous system. Think of it as a kind of behavioral confusion. Apraxic patients may have difficulty getting dressed in the morning because they have forgotten how to button clothes or tie shoes. Or they may have problems driving correctly, whereas in that past, driving was taken for granted. The best way to determine if this has been a problem is by asking family members questions such as

> *Does your father have problems getting dressed on his own?*
> *Does he need any help with shaving or putting on a tie?*
> *Can he throw a sandwich together easily?*

You can sometimes assess apraxia during the interview by observing your patient doing something (e.g., pulling her hospital registration card from her wallet), or you can ask the patient to write down your office phone number and observe her ability to procure a piece of paper and pen and correctly write down the number.

The Folstein MMSE includes a standard three-step command for assessing apraxia:

> *Now I want to see how well you can follow instructions. I'm going to give you a piece of paper. Take it in your right hand, use both hands to fold it in half, then put it on the floor.*

6. **Social cognition.** This is DSM-5's jargon for what we sometimes call "personality changes." As dementia develops and worsens, patients have problems reading social cues and behaving appropriately. They may withdraw from conversations or bring up awkward things, like topics relating to sex, politics, or religion. You may observe this in your conversation with your patient, and you can ask informants if this has become a problem.

Assessing Eating Disorders and Somatic Symptom Disorder

Screening Questions
- Eating disorders: Have you ever thought you had an eating disorder, like anorexia or bulimia?
- Somatic symptom disorder: Do you worry a lot about your health?

EATING DISORDERS

KEY POINT

Eating disorders are relatively easily diagnosed (Tables 29.1, 29.2, and 29.3). The problem is that many clinicians don't ask about them, and many sufferers don't volunteer their symptoms, either because they aren't bothered by them, as in anorexia, or because they're too ashamed of them, as in bulimia and binge eating disorder. Therefore, screening questions for eating disorders should always be included in your PROS.

When time is truly of the essence, you can begin with a direct question:

Have you ever had an eating disorder, such as anorexia or bulimia?

However, if you have the sense that your patient may be particularly ashamed of a suspected eating disorder, a too blunt approach might endanger the therapeutic alliance. In these cases, you can approach the issue more indirectly:

Have you ever thought you were overweight?

If the answer is "no," it is unlikely that your patient has an either anorexia or bulimia. If the answer is yes, and you suspect anorexia, ask:

TABLE 29.1. *DSM-5* **Criteria for Anorexia Nervosa**

Mnemonic: **W**eight **F**ear **B**others Anorexics
  Weight significantly low
  Intense **F**ear of gaining weight or becoming fat
  Distorted **B**ody image

Adapted from American Psychiatric Association. (2013). *Diagnostic and Statistical Manual of Mental Disorders*, 5th ed. Washington, DC: American Psychiatric Association.

Have you ever dieted?

Almost everyone, and women in particular, has dieted at some point. You're probing here for a particularly severe diet, perhaps a starvation diet (i.e., fasting) or a diet in which, for example, the patient ate only salad or fruit.

Have you ever weighed much less than people thought you should weigh? What was your lowest weight? And what is your height?

You want to determine what your patient's lowest body mass index (BMI) was. The BMI is calculated as a person's weight in kilograms divided by the height in meters squared. There are plenty of free online BMI calculators. While DSM-IV required that a patient's weight be no more than 85% of the ideal body weight to qualify for anorexia, that's no longer the case with DSM-5. Instead, there are suggested BMI benchmarks to help you to judge the severity of the disorder, which are printed in the DSM-5.

Did you think you were overweight at your lowest weight?

Anorexic patients will report feeling overweight, even obese, at a weight that is far below their ideal weight. Often,

TABLE 29.2. *DSM-5* **Criteria for Bulimia Nervosa**

Mnemonic: **B**ulimics **O**ver-**C**onsume **P**astries
  Recurrent episodes of **B**inge eating (at least once a week for 3 mo) that feel **O**ut of control
  Excessive **C**oncern with body shape and weight
  Purging behaviors, such as self-induced vomiting; misuse of laxatives, diuretics, enemas, or other medications; fasting; or excessive exercise

Adapted from American Psychiatric Association. (2013). *Diagnostic and Statistical Manual of Mental Disorders*, 5th ed. Washington, DC: American Psychiatric Association.

TABLE 29.3. *DSM-5* **Criteria for Binge Eating Disorder**

Recurrent episodes of binge eating (at least once a week for 3 mo) that feel out of control (required)

One or more of the following must be associated with the binge eating episodes:

Eating very quickly, eating to the point feeling painfully full, eating when not really hungry, eating alone because of feeling embarrassed about the behavior, feeling disgusted with oneself afterward.

Adapted from American Psychiatric Association. (2013). *Diagnostic and Statistical Manual of Mental Disorders*, 5th ed. Washington, DC: American Psychiatric Association.

the patient will fixate on a particular body part, such as the thighs or the stomach.

> *Were you afraid of gaining weight?*

For both bulimia and binge eating disorder (BED), good screening questions are:

> *Have you ever felt like your eating was out of control? Do you have eating binges when you eat a large amount of food than you should and feel like you can't stop eating?*

 TIP

You have to be somewhat skeptical of a "yes" answer, because what the patient considers a binge may seem like a normal meal to someone else. Ask your patient to describe the contents of a typical binge and decide whether it seems like an unusually large meal.

If she binges, ask if she has ever purged afterward.

> *After you've binged, have you ever gotten rid of the food in some way, such as vomiting or taking laxatives?*

Establish the frequency of the behavior with a symptom exaggeration question:

> *At the most, how often were you binging and purging? Once a day? Twice a day? More?*

If the patient has binged but has never purged, then you should ask some or all of the following questions to rule in or out BED.

> *Tell me a little more about your binging. Do you eat quickly? Do you eat to the point of feeling too full? Do you binge alone? Do you feel bad about yourself afterward? Do you ever binge even though you're not hungry?*

SOMATIC SYMPTOM DISORDER AND ILLNESS ANXIETY DISORDER

In DSM-IV, somatization disorder, or hypochondriasis, was used to diagnose patients who worried excessively about multiple somatic symptoms—which were medically unexplained. DSM-5 has abolished somatization disorder, substituting two different diagnoses, which differ in subtle ways:

> *Somatic symptom disorder (SSD) refers to people who have actual somatic symptoms (which may or may not be caused by an established medical problem) but who are so excessively preoccupied with the symptoms that they have problems functioning (Table 29.4).*
> *Illness anxiety disorder refers to people who do not actually have somatic symptoms but who are extremely worried that they have an illness—in the absence of any medical evidence that they do (Table 29.5).*

TABLE 29.4. *DSM-5* Criteria for Somatic Symptom Disorder

There is one or more somatic symptom that has been persistent for at least 6 mo and that may or may not have an established medical origin.

The patient has been overly focused on the symptom(s), as defined by one or more of the following:

Excessive thoughts about the seriousness of the symptom

High levels of anxiety about the symptom

Too much time devoted to thinking about or responding to the symptom

Adapted from American Psychiatric Association. (2013). *Diagnostic and Statistical Manual of Mental Disorders*, 5th ed. Washington, DC: American Psychiatric Association.

TABLE 29.5. *DSM-5* Criteria for Illness Anxiety Disorder

The patient believes he or she has a serious illness but it has not been diagnosed and there are no accompanying symptoms (or if there are they are milder than what you'd expect for the illness.)

For at least 6 months the patient has been highly anxious about the illness and has spent excessive amounts of time or energy focusing on it.

Adapted from American Psychiatric Association. (2013). *Diagnostic and Statistical Manual of Mental Disorders*, 5th ed. Washington, DC: American Psychiatric Association.

For either disorder, an excellent screening question is

> *Do you tend to worry a lot about your health?*

If the patient says "no," you can avoid the probing questions. If he says yes, proceed as below. In truth, a patient with either disorder will have likely already hinted at the problem when you elicited the history of present illness (HPI), much of which will have been devoted to discussions of health issues.

Your next job is to determine if there are any actual symptoms.

> *You mentioned that you worry about your health. What health issues are you worrying about? What kinds of symptoms do you have?*

The patient with SSD will launch into a list of somatic symptoms, like pain, fatigue, diarrhea, palpitations, and the like. On the other hand, the patient with anxiety illness disorder will not provide much information about specific symptoms and will instead say something like: "It's pretty vague, I just know I'm sick and I'm pretty sure it's cancer."

As you can see, it can be hard to differentiate between these two conditions. Generally, patients who used to qualify for "somatization disorder" (which required at least seven discrete somatic symptoms) will likely be diagnosed with new disorder, SSD. Patients with the new illness anxiety disorder may describe some symptoms as well, but the symptoms will be described more vaguely and there won't be as many of them.

The somatic disorders were reorganized in this way not in order to confuse us—though that will surely happen. The major impetus was to remove some of the stigma that has become attached to somatization disorder and the derogatory label "hypochondriac." Such patients are often made to feel that their symptoms are "all in their head," when in fact they actually *do* perceive symptoms, along with an overlay of anxiety that makes the symptoms feel worse.

Assessing Attention Deficit Hyperactivity Disorder

30

Screening Question
- When you were young, did you have problems with hyperactivity or with paying attention in school?

ATTENTION DEFICIT HYPERACTIVITY DISORDER

Patients must meet either criterion 1 or criterion 2 (must have six of nine disorganization/inattention symptoms or six of nine impulsivity/hyperactivity symptoms—but for those aged 17 or older, the threshold number of symptoms is lowered to five of nine) plus criteria 3 and 4 (Table 30.1):

1. Organization/inattention
   Organization problems
   - Can't organize tasks
   - Loses things needed for tasks
   - Has problems finishing tasks
   Attention problems
   - Poor focus
   - Easily distracted
   - Doesn't listen
   - Forgets easily
   - Makes careless mistakes
   - Avoids tasks requiring concentration
2. Impulsivity/hyperactivity symptoms
   - Talks too much
   - Blurts out answers
   - Interrupts others
   - Can't play quietly
   Movement excess
   - Fidgets and squirms
   - Leaves seat

TABLE 30.1. *DSM-5* Criteria for Attention Deficit Hyperactivity Disorder

Mnemonic: You'll need a **MOAT** around the classroom for the hyperactive child.

    Movement excess (hyperactivity)
    Organization problems (difficulty finishing tasks)
    Attention problems
    Talking impulsively

Data from American Psychiatric Association. (2013). Diagnostic and Statistical Manual of Mental Disorders, 5th ed. Washington, DC: American Psychiatric Association.

- Is restless
- Is on the go
- Can't wait for his turn
3. Some symptoms must have been present before age 12.
4. Symptoms occur in two or more settings, such as school (or work) and at home.

ADHD is one of those disorders, such as panic disorder, that involve a long list of criteria, making it impractical to memorize each one. To make matters more confusing, many of the criteria are so similar as to be redundant (e.g., is there really a difference between "often fails to pay close attention" and "often has difficulty sustaining attention"?). Therefore, as was true for panic disorder, the most rational approach is to clump criteria into meaningful clusters by using a mnemonic, in this case MOAT.

To meet the criteria, your patient must have six of nine symptoms of inattention/disorganization *or* six of nine symptoms of hyperactivity/impulsivity.

ATTENTION DEFICIT HYPERACTIVITY DISORDER IN CHILDREN

Although it may seem counterintuitive, diagnosing ADHD is generally easier in children than in adults. This is because children and adolescents come to the appointment with an adult who is (hopefully) a reliable source of behavioral information. Also, one of the key difficulties in establishing the diagnosis in adults is documenting that symptoms occurred as a child; this is a nonissue when you have a living, breathing child in front of you!

For tips on evaluating adolescent patients, review Chapter 10. Generally, you'll begin your evaluation with family in the room. The parents have brought their child to you for an ADHD evaluation, so get right down to it:

> *So what makes you think Johnny has ADHD?*

Parents will often come bearing testing reports from the school and will also often have misconceptions about how easy (or hard) the condition is to diagnose. ("We're not sure whether or not Johnny has ADHD, and we were hoping you could test him for it. Do you do testing here?")

Now it's time for some basic psychoeducation about ADHD. The diagnosis is based on a synthesis of different people's reports and observations of the child, and there is no definitive "test" apart from good interviewing and deduction.

> *What we'll do today is talk about Johnny's behavior, both at home and at school, and based on that, we'll come up with a good idea of whether he has ADHD.*

The essence of the diagnosis is asking about all the *DSM-5* criteria, and the approach that works best for me is to simply photocopy the *DSM-5* criteria for the parents and patient to look over, and to go down the list, asking about each one in turn. You can read the criteria verbatim, or you can paraphrase it to make it more understandable, depending on the sophistication of your informants.

For example, for organization problems, you would say something like

> *Does Johnny not pay close attention to details, or does he make careless mistakes at school or at home?*

For each criterion, I try to establish not only that it happens but that it happens in two different settings, and I also ask for a specific example to assess how significant the symptom is. I recommend writing all these examples down; later, after treatment has begun, it's very helpful to go through all these examples to assess how much better things are than before you worked your treatment magic!

Once you are done, you can say:

> *Well, it looks like Johnny definitely meets diagnostic criteria for ADHD, because as you can see, he has almost all the symptoms listed here.*

Occasionally, you'll be able to observe blatant hyperactivity (12-year-old tearing around your office, causing damage to the cherished painted giraffe you bought in Oaxaca), but usually not. Certainly, if the patient has ADD without the "H," it's very hard to notice poor focus in a highly charged and focused setting like a psychiatric office.

KEY POINT

As you ask the *DSM-5* questions, remember that many psychiatric disorders other than ADHD can cause problems of impulsivity or concentration, including substance abuse, depression, mania, and anxiety disorders (Biederman 1991). If a child meets only a few ADHD criteria but is still causing the parents' conniption fits, move your questioning to these other diagnostic categories.

ATTENTION DEFICIT HYPERACTIVITY DISORDER IN ADULTS

Adult ADHD has become quite the rage in recent years. Some days, it seems that every other patient entering your office ends up wondering if they should try methylphenidate (Ritalin), which seems to work so well for their son or daughter. Unfortunately, it is easy to feign symptoms of ADHD, and one study found that a quarter of adult patients either feigned or exaggerated ADHD symptoms, presumably in order to get a prescription for stimulants, which are highly abusable (Marshall et al. 2010).

DSM-5 made it easier for adults to qualify for the diagnosis in two ways: first, the required onset of symptoms was moved from age 7 to age 12; second, the minimum threshold of required symptoms was lowered from 6 to 5 for adults but not for kids. For tips on figuring out if a patient is malingering, review Chapter 9.

As usual, begin with some screening questions:

> *When you were in elementary or junior high school, did you have problems with hyperactivity or paying attention in class?*

If the response is positive, ask

> *Do you still have those sorts of problems?*

If the answer is negative, it's probably not worth your time to continue with probing questions to verify an old diagnosis of ADHD. If the answer is positive, move on to questions establishing the diagnosis. You can whip out the *DSM-5* criteria as was recommended above, or you can ask questions in a less structured fashion, starting first with questions pertaining to inattentiveness and then moving on to questions about impulsivity.

Inattentiveness and Disorganization

> *Do you have a hard time paying attention to things?*
> *Do you have trouble concentrating?*

Some patients find that they are able to concentrate on engaging tasks, such as watching a football game or reading a tabloid, but not on tasks that are less fun, such as writing a report at work or studying for school.

> *Are you distractible?*

Because many people will not know what this means, you might need to follow up with

> *Do you know what that means? It means that you can't listen to the teacher if the guy next to you is talking or if something's happening outside the window.*
> *Do you have a hard time finishing things?*

Some patients may not think of their problem as inattentiveness, but they do find that they get distracted in the middle of a task and don't finish projects. If the patient's parent is present, ask

> *Was he the type of kid who, if you said, "Go to your room and get your shoes," wouldn't come back because he got interested in something else and forgot about the shoes?*

Talking Impulsively and Hyperactivity

> *Were you the class clown?*

The typical ADHD patient will break into a smile and say, "Oh yeah, let me tell you…" and may describe some choice antics. A variation on this question is

> *When you were in class, was the teacher always having to say to you, "Now, Johnny, you need to stop doing this or that"?*

Some patients will say that they are hyperactive when what they mean is overly energetic, as in a manic episode, or anxious. Ask your patient for his definition:

> *What do you mean when you say that you're hyperactive?*

Provide your own definition, if necessary:

> *By hyperactive, I mean a feeling that you can't sit still, almost as though you had a little motor running inside you all the time that you can't turn off.*

Other specific questions to ask include

> *Do you have a hard time keeping still?*
> *Do you tend to be fidgety?*

Although hyperactivity in children may be observable during an initial session, in adolescents and adults it presents more subtly. You may observe constant foot tapping or rapid hand gestures. The personality style will often be characteristic—outgoing, chatty, and lively—although these are hardly diagnostic of ADHD and are reminiscent of mania.

To ask about impulsive talking, a good question is

> *Is it easy for you to sit quietly at meetings or in class, or do you tend to blurt things out a lot?*

Formal Rating Scales and Family Interviews

Interviewing a patient's parents (even when the patient is an adult) will always make an ADHD diagnosis easier. Often, the parent will say, "Oh yes, he was diagnosed with ADHD in school," and will brandish psychological test reports.

The most common rating scale is the Conners' Scale, available through school systems and in most institutional child psychiatry departments. If a parent or spouse is present, complete the scale with him during the initial visit. In addition, give the patient a copy to take home to be filled out by a teacher or employer. Remember that you have to establish that your patient's symptoms occur in at least two different settings to make the diagnosis of ADHD.

Assessing Personality Disorders

> **Essential Concepts**
> - Use the ground-up technique to assess for PDs from the social history.
> - Use the symptom-window technique to assess for PDs that might be linked to specific symptoms.
> - Memorize self-statements, probing questions, and mnemonics for each disorder.

The *DSM-5* emphasizes the medical model of psychiatric disorders. Each disorder is presented as though it was a discrete syndrome that a patient "has," in the same way that she might "have" diabetes or asthma. Most clinicians realize that this is a simplistic view and understand that each patient has an underlying personality that interacts and often contributes to the formation of a psychiatric syndrome. Earlier versions of DSM included an "Axis II," which was specifically for personality disorders (PDs), and served the useful function of forcing to at least give some thought to every client's personality traits. While DSM-5 eliminated the diagnostic axes, it still goes to great lengths describing PDs and includes a new section on an alternative model for PDs. While interesting, this model is complex and still under review and is not something you need to know (yet) in evaluating your patients.

PDs are notoriously difficult to diagnose. It is the rare clinician who can confidently conclude after a single interview that a patient has a PD. Thus, this chapter does not assume that you will be able to diagnose a PD quickly, but rather that you will be able to formulate some good hypotheses. Such hypotheses are usually noted in the chart as "rule out_____ personality disorder."

TWO GENERAL APPROACHES

Two general strategies are useful for assessing PDs in the interview. They are not mutually exclusive, and clinicians commonly use both over the course of the evaluation.

Strategy 1: The Ground-Up Technique

In the ground-up technique, you gradually fashion a picture of your patient's personality by working from the ground up—that is, by learning about her life history chronologically in the context of the social and family history. As outlined in Chapter 18, the formal social history often begins with a general question about family life.

> *Tell me a bit about what growing up was like for you.*

As you ask chronologic questions about your patient's life, especially those aspects of life that involve interpersonal relationships, try to identify any dysfunctional patterns of relating. Recurrent patterns are the hallmark of PDs. Memorize one or two probing questions for each PD (see the following examples) and ask them at appropriate times.

A typical example is the patient who relates a pattern of having had few close friendships throughout the early years of his life. Depending on the patient's behavior toward you during the interview (see the section on Behavioral Clues), you may have some hypotheses about which PD is most likely. Perhaps, the patient appears anxious and shy during the interview, leading you to suspect avoidant PD. You would then ask a probing question, such as

> *Have you tended to have few friends in your life because you didn't want to have friends, or because you were scared of getting close to someone who might reject you?*

Using the ground-up technique, you will usually be able to arrive at a good hypothesis for a PD or personality traits.

Consider the following example.

CLINICAL VIGNETTE

The interviewer is asking a patient about his work history:

> *Interviewer: What sorts of jobs have you had?*
> *Patient: I've had a whole bunch of different jobs. I don't stick with any one job for very long.*
> *Interviewer: What usually happens with these jobs?*
> *Patient: I usually quit, because the people I work with end up backstabbing me.*

At this point, the interviewer suspects paranoid PD and asks the probing questions.

Interviewer: Have you found in your life that people have turned against you for no good reason?
Patient: Yeah, beginning with my parents.
Interviewer: Do you tend to think of people in general as being disloyal or dishonest?
Patient: Well, I've found that you just can't trust anyone, because they'll always try to do you in if you let down your guard.

The interviewer, having established two of the four criteria required to make the diagnosis of paranoid PD, will then go on to ask questions regarding other criteria.

Strategy 2: The Symptom-Window Technique

The symptom-window technique entails beginning with your patient's major symptoms and using them as "windows" for exploring possible roots in PDs. This is generally done toward the end of the past psychiatric history (PPH), by which time you will have identified the major symptoms and delineated the syndromal and treatment history. The next step is to ask questions about events that may have occurred each time the symptoms arose. Were these interpersonal events? Were they related to life transitions? In your judgment, do the symptoms seem to be reasonable responses to the events, or do they seem exaggerated?

The nature of the symptoms per se does little to point to a specific PD, but using the symptoms as windows to the personality is often productive. For example, a major depression can be a product of virtually any of the PDs, but each patient will arrive at the depression by a different route. Here are some typical examples:

- Narcissistic PD: The patient finds that nobody meets his high standards, thereby alienating friends and family, leading to a social isolation that can cause depression.
- Avoidant PD: The patient avoids friendships for fear of rejection, leading to loneliness and depression.
- Dependent PD: Patient develops a sense of worthlessness and demoralization because of an inability to make life decisions without relying on someone else.

- Borderline PD: A chronic sense of inner emptiness may lead to depression, suicidality, and other problems, such as substance abuse, bulimia, and impulse control disorder.

As an example, assume you are interviewing a patient with major depression who recently considered overdosing on some medication after being rejected by her boyfriend. You suspect borderline PD. You can broach the issue with a referred transition:

> *Earlier, we were talking about your depression and some of the suicidal thoughts you had after your boyfriend left you. Have you reacted in this way to rejection at other times in your life?*

After you've gotten the ball rolling by using the referred transition, you can run through the rest of the criteria, jogging your memory with the mnemonic I DESPAIRR. You can introduce these questions with a remark such as

> *I'd like to ask a few more questions about your personality and the ways that you tend to react to certain situations. I'm interested in learning about what sort of person you've been since your teenage years, not only how you've been over the last few weeks.*

This helps to ensure that your patient answers in terms of enduring personality traits rather than recent symptoms.

◆ KEY POINT

This last point deserves repeating: A PD refers to a *persisting* pattern of dysfunctional relating styles *over many years*, at least since adolescence or young adulthood. Thus, when you ask about criteria for a PD, make clear to your patient that you're interested in the long-term view. Beginners often forget this and may end up falsely diagnosing a PD when the patient actually has an acute Axis I disorder. For example, depressed patients commonly appear irritable, needy, and suicidal, features that could easily lead to the diagnosis of borderline PD. Once the depression clears, such patients may magically shed their Axis II pathology.

SPECIFIC PERSONALITY DISORDERS: SELF-STATEMENTS, PROBING QUESTIONS, AND BEHAVIORAL CLUES

I have listed below all 10 *DSM-5* PDs. For each, there is a patient "self-statement," which is a hypothetical description that a patient with the given disorder would make about himself. The statements are simplistic and stereotypic and are only meant to be used as memory aids, so that you can dependably fix the main features of each PD in your mind. Two suggested probing questions, along with common behavioral clues that might increase your suspicion of a particular disorder, are listed beneath each statement. Finally, a mnemonic is given for each PD, all of which (except the one for borderline PD) were written by Harold Pinkofsky (1997). If you obtain positive responses to your probing questions, follow up with more questions related to specific diagnostic criteria, using the mnemonics as aids. As an illustration, I have included questions that can be used for each of the criteria for borderline PD.

Borderline Personality Disorder

- Self-statement: "I need people desperately, and when people reject me I fall apart completely. I hate them, and I get suicidal."
- Probing questions:

    Have people often disappointed you in your life?
    When something has gone really wrong in your life, such as losing a job or getting rejected, have you often done something to hurt yourself, such as cutting yourself or overdosing?

- Behavioral clues: May alternatively idealize and devalue you over the course of the interview; may be unusually emotionally labile.

Mnemonic: **I DESPAIRR**

Identity disturbance

    Have you generally been pretty clear about what your goals are in life and what sort of person you are, or do you have trouble knowing who_____is? (Say patient's name.)

Disordered, unstable affect owing to a marked reactivity of mood

> *Are you a moody person?*

Chronic feelings of Emptiness

> *Do you often feel empty inside?*

Recurrent Suicidal behavior, gestures, or threats, or self-mutilating behavior

> *Looking back, when something has gone really wrong in your life, like losing a job or getting rejected, have you often done something to hurt yourself, such as cutting or overdosing?*

Transient, stress-related Paranoid ideation or severe dissociative symptoms

> *When you're under stress, do you feel you lose touch with your environment or with yourself? During those times, do you feel as if people are ganging up on you?*

Frantic efforts to avoid real or imagined Abandonment

> *When someone abandons or rejects you, how do you react?*

Impulsivity in at least two areas that is potentially self-damaging

> *Do you see yourself as an overly impulsive person?*
> *Have you ever done things that can get you into trouble, such as spending all your money, driving like a maniac, using a lot of drugs, having a lot of sex, and so forth?*

Inappropriate, intense Rage or difficulty controlling anger

> *What do you do when you get angry?*
> *Do you hold it inside or let loose with it so that everybody knows how you're feeling?*

A pattern of unstable and intense interpersonal Relationships characterized by alternating extremes of idealization and devaluation

> *Do your relationships tend to be calm and stable or stormy and unstable, with lots of ups and downs?*

Cluster A ("Odd")

Paranoid

- Self-statement: "Others are untrustworthy, and they try to take advantage of me."
- Probing questions:

  Have you often found that people in your life have not been trustworthy?
  Have people turned against you for no good reason?

- Behavioral clues: Patient appears guarded and suspicious; patient answers questions reluctantly and with an air of suspicion.

Mnemonic: **SUSPECT** (four of these seven)

Spousal infidelity suspected
Unforgiving (bears grudges)
Suspicious of others
Perceives attacks
Views everyone as either an Enemy or a friend
Confiding in others feared
Threats perceived in benign events

Schizoid

- Self-statement: "I prefer to be alone; my world is completely empty."
- Probing questions:

  Are you a people person, or are you someone who prefers to be alone? (Prefers to be alone.)
  Can you name some things that you really enjoy doing? (Takes pleasure in few, if any, activities.)

- Behavioral clues: Patient appears shy and aloof. Patient seems to be preoccupied, in her own world.

Mnemonic: **DISTANT** (four of these seven)

Detached (or flattened) affect
Indifferent to criticism or praise
Sexual experiences of little interest
Tasks (activities) performed solitarily
Absence of close friends
Neither desires nor enjoys close relations
Takes pleasure in few activities

Schizotypal

- Self-statement: "I'd like to have friends but it's hard, because people find me pretty strange."
- Probing questions:

  Do you tend to feel pretty uncomfortable around other people?

  Do you sometimes have ideas that other people don't really understand or find unusual?

  Behavioral clues: Patient appears odd in any number of ways—for example, she may be disheveled, wearing strange clothes, or have odd mannerisms. Patient describes strange ideas that border on psychotic.

Mnemonic: **ME PECULIAR** (five of first nine plus "rule out" specifier)

Magical thinking or odd beliefs
Experiences unusual perceptions
Paranoid ideation
Eccentric behavior or appearance
Constricted (or inappropriate) affect
Unusual (odd) thinking and speech
Lacks close friends
Ideas of reference
Anxiety in social situations
Rule out psychotic disorder and autistic disorder

Cluster B ("Dramatic")

Borderline

See the earlier Borderline Section.

Antisocial

- Self-statement: "I love to take advantage of other people, and I never feel bad about it."
- Probing questions:

  Do you admire a good scam when you see it?

  Have you ever done anything that could have gotten you in trouble with the law?

- Behavioral clues: The patient is excessively cocky and arrogant. The patient always portrays self as innocent and a victim in violent or criminal circumstances.

Mnemonic: **CORRUPT** (three of these seven)

Conformity to law lacking
Obligations ignored
Reckless disregard for safety of self or others
Remorse lacking
Underhanded (deceitful, lies, cons others)
Planning insufficient (impulsive)
Temper

Histrionic

- Self-statement: "I'm quite an emotional and sexually charming person, and I need to be the center of attention!"
- Probing questions:

  Do you like to be the center of attention? (Yes.)
  When you feel an emotion, do you keep it inside or do you express it? (Express it.)

- Behavioral clues: The patient is flamboyantly and seductively groomed or dressed. The patient is rapidly and dramatically self-revealing to the point of inappropriateness, even in the context of a psychiatric evaluation.

Mnemonic: **PRAISE ME** (five of these eight)

Provocative (or sexually seductive) behavior
Relationships (considered more intimate than they are)
Attention (uncomfortable when not the center of attention)
Influenced easily
Style of speech (impressionistic, lacks detail)
Emotions (rapidly shifting and shallow)
Made up (physical appearance used to draw attention to self)
Emotions exaggerated (theatrical)

Narcissistic

- Self-statement: "I'm an extremely talented and special person, better than most people, and yet I get angry and depressed because people don't recognize how great I am!"

- Probing questions:

  Do you often find yourself getting frustrated because other people don't meet your standards? (Yes.)
  What are your ambitions for yourself? (Will be unrealistically high.)

- Behavioral clues: The patient may appear haughty and excessively critical of your credentials or experience. She may begin the interview with a litany of angry complaints about how unfairly others have treated her.

Mnemonic: **SPEEECIAL** (five of these nine)

Special (believes he is special and unique)
Preoccupied with fantasies (e.g., of unlimited success, power)
Envious
Entitlement
Excessive admiration required
Conceited
Interpersonal exploitation
Arrogant
Lacks empathy

Cluster C ("Anxious")

Avoidant

- Self-statement: "I'm really afraid of what people will think of me, so I avoid making new friends to prevent rejection."
- Probing questions:

  Do you tend to avoid meeting people or getting close to people? (Yes.)
  Is that because you prefer to be alone or because you've been rejected before and you don't want it to happen again? (The latter.)

- Behavioral clues: The patient may appear shy and nervous but with a poignant eagerness to make contact. He may begin the interview reluctant to open up and will typically become quite self-revealing once rapport has been established.

Mnemonic: **CRINGES** (four of these seven)

Certainty of being liked required before willing to risk involvement

Rejection possibility preoccupies his thoughts
Intimate relationships avoided
New relationships avoided
Gets around occupational activities that involve interpersonal contact
Embarrassment potential prevents new activities
Self viewed as unappealing, inept, inferior

Dependent

- Self-statement: "I'm pretty passive and dependent on others for direction, and I go far out of my way not to displease people who are important to me."
- Probing questions:

  Do you consider yourself a completely independent person, or have you tended to lean on others in your life for emotional support and guidance? (Lean on someone else.) Who has made most major decisions in your life, you or your_____ (spouse, parents, or other, depending on situation)? (Someone other than the patient.)

- Behavioral clues: The patient will seem to make extraordinary attempts to immediately gain your affection.

  Mnemonic: **RELIANCE** (five of these eight)

  Reassurance required for decisions
  Expressing disagreement difficult (because of fear of loss of support or approval)
  Life responsibilities assumed by others
  Initiating projects difficult
  Alone (feels helpless and a sense of discomfort when alone)
  Nurturance (goes to excessive lengths to obtain nurturance and support)
  Companionship sought urgently when close relationship ends
  Exaggerated fears of being left to care for self

Obsessive-Compulsive

- Self-statement: "I'm a perfectionist. I keep lists, I drive myself hard, and I'm very serious about life."
- Probing questions:

  *Do you consider yourself a perfectionist?
  Do you drive yourself so hard with your work that you find you have no time for leisure activities?*

- Behavioral clues: The patient is meticulously groomed and dressed. He will tend to give an excessively detailed and accurate account of his symptoms.

Mnemonic: **LAW FIRMS** (four of these eight)

Loses point of activity
Ability to complete tasks compromised by perfectionism
Worthless objects (unable to discard)
Friendships (and leisure activities) excluded (owing to preoccupation with work)
Inflexible, scrupulous, overconscientious
Reluctant to delegate
Miserly
Stubborn

IV

INTERVIEWING FOR TREATMENT

How to Educate Your Patient

Does this mean I'm crazy?
Is this medication going to turn me into a zombie?
Am I going to be this way for the rest of my life?

These are the sorts of questions that patients will ask you, often toward the end of the diagnostic interview. Clinicians eventually develop an effective approach to answering such questions in lay terms. Although patient education is rarely formally taught in training programs, from the patient's perspective, it is often the most important part of the initial evaluation.

Educating your patient about his disorder is helpful for various reasons. First, education decreases his anxiety. As clinicians, we tend to take mental illness for granted, but patients are often terrified by their disorders. By giving an illness a name and showing that its prognosis and treatment are well understood and that millions of other people have experienced it, we can significantly decrease the patient's anxiety.

Second, patient education improves adherence to treatment, both for medications and for therapy. Misconceptions about psychiatric treatment abound in our society; most people get their information about psychiatry from television shows, newspapers, and the Internet, which leads to a mismatch between reality and fantasy. For example, many patients believe that psychotherapy is a long-term process in which painful family dynamics are rehashed for years on end. Such a misconception decreases the likelihood that patients will commit to therapy. When educated about the fact that most present-day therapy is brief and focuses on current problems, patients become more receptive to referrals.

Misinformation about medications also abounds. Patients often believe that antidepressants are to be discontinued once they feel better, as opposed to the 6 to 12 months of continuous therapy recommended. Other patients consider antidepressants to be rapid mood boosters. One patient for whom I had prescribed Prozac for depression came back in a month reporting that she had only "needed to take" the Prozac four or five times. Her belief had been that the medication was to be taken only on those mornings that she awoke feeling very depressed.

In this chapter, I guide you through a commonly used strategy for providing patient education that can be applied to a wide variety of mental disorders.

BRIEFLY STATE YOUR DIAGNOSIS

Although this is self-explanatory, I would add that you needn't always phrase the diagnosis in *DSM-5* terminology. For example, I often tell patients that they have a "clinical depression" rather than a "major depression," because I know from experience that more patients have heard of the former than the latter.

WHAT YOUR PATIENT KNOWS ABOUT THE DISORDER

The way I generally find out what my patient knows about the disorder is as an extension of providing a diagnosis. Thus:

> *I think that you've been suffering from a clinical, or major, depression. Do you know what that is?*

If the patient says "yes," I ask him to elaborate a bit:

> *What is your definition of depression?*

As a prelude to treatment negotiation, I often ask whether the patient has any expectations about treatment.

> *Do you have any ideas about treatment?*

Some patients may overtly request a particular form of treatment, such as psychotherapy or medication, whereas others may tell you what they *don't* want.

MINILECTURE ABOUT THE DISORDER

Not all patients want to hear you wax poetic about their disorders. For example, a well-informed patient who has just delineated each of the *DSM-5* criteria of OCD might be insulted to hear you repeat them. Other patients may be quite uninformed but, taking the attitude that you, and not they, are the doctor, might feel uncomfortable with your efforts to educate them and involve them in their treatment. There's no firm rule about which patients should get a minilecture. Accordingly, you can ask the patient something like this:

> *Would you like me to give you some information on depression?*

Although it is the rare patient who responds with a flat "no," even if he'd prefer not to have the information, you can generally gauge the degree of interest based on the response and adjust the length of your minilecture accordingly.

As a guide for structuring your minilecture, I turn to the experience of the researchers at the University of Pittsburgh, who used a psychoeducational program that helped them achieve a remarkably high (90%) adherence to treatment over 3 years (Frank et al. 1995; Jacobs et al. 1987). Their program was devised to teach patients and their families about depression. Its components included the following:

- Define the illness. Ask your patient to identify all the symptoms that he has experienced. A chalkboard, or, more realistically, a piece of paper on which to write, is helpful. Define the disorder as an illness that has many symptoms, including the ones your patient has identified; try to portray it as an illness similar to the medical illnesses of diabetes or hypertension. This helps decrease the stigma associated with mental illness.
- Discuss the prevalence and course of the illness. (Refer to Appendix A for a pocket card listing the prevalence for the major mental disorders.)
- Discuss the causes. Although we don't know the causes of most mental illnesses, you can discuss some different theories.
- Discuss the options for treatment.
- For medications, discuss side effect profiles and emphasize the fact that individuals experience different side effects. Over the past decade, a larger proportion of

psychiatric visits have involved medication management, and we are often confronted with patients who are ambivalent about taking the treatments we prescribe. As Shea (2006) points out in his excellent book on medication adherence, a helpful trick for prodding reluctant patients into considering medications is to borrow a pediatrician's technique called "inquiry into lost dreams." As quoted in Shea's book, "I find it useful with my kids with asthma to ask them this question or a variation of it, 'Is there anything that your asthma is keeping you from doing that you really wish you could do again?' What I find with this age group is that there is often a quick answer to this question, and the answer is often related to a sport, say, football or soccer."

You can readily adopt this technique to psychiatric issues: "Is there anything that your anxiety is keeping you from doing that you wish you could do again?" The answer may help your patient better appreciate the potential benefits of medications.

Here is an example of a minilecture for major depression:

> *A major depression is a breakdown in a person's ability to cope with stress. While we all get sad from time to time when things go poorly, a person with major depression feels so down that the basic functions of living are affected. As with medical illnesses, depression causes specific symptoms. In your case, you haven't been able to sleep, you've lost your appetite, you haven't been able to concentrate at work, and you've had some scary suicidal thoughts.*
>
> *Depression is quite common; about 10% of people develop it at some point in their lives. What causes it isn't clear. For some people, stressors seem to cause depression; this may be the case for you, since you felt bad after your divorce. In other cases, depression seems to be a biologic disorder.*
>
> *The good news about depression is that it's very treatable. There are two main techniques, medication or talk therapy. A combination of the two is often most effective. In your case, I'd recommend the combined treatment. Do you have any questions about all this?*

I'll also give you an example of a minilecture for borderline personality disorders, just to prove that you can discuss personality disorders with patients without sounding critical.

I: *You're suffering from borderline personality disorder. Do you know what that is?*

P: *No, but it sounds bad, like being on the edge.*

I: *You're not far off. It is a bit like being on the edge. People with borderline personality disorder tend to have poor self-esteem, and this causes them to be very moody, especially when it comes to dealing with friends and family. For instance, you told me earlier that when people reject you, you don't just get depressed, you get suicidal. And when you get angry at people, you really lose control.*

P: *That's just the way I've always been; I didn't know it was an official disorder.*

I: *It is, and believe me, you're not alone. Studies show that about 2% of all people have the same problem. No one knows exactly what causes it, but the early family environment usually plays a role. The best treatment is long-term therapy, with medications from time to time to treat depression.*

You'll develop your own style of educating patients, and your lecture will inevitably vary depending on the patient. As much as possible, you want to speak your patient's language, which will vary with level of intelligence and education, cultural background, age, and other factors.

QUESTIONS

Even if you are feeling the pressure of the end of the hour, give your patient plenty of time to think about questions.

WRITTEN EDUCATIONAL MATERIALS

Giving written educational materials to your patients allows them to consider the information in privacy and at greater length. You may use the handouts in Appendix B, all of which are public domain documents that can be reproduced with or without acknowledgments.

Negotiating a Treatment Plan

Essential Concepts
- Elicit the patient's agenda.
- Negotiate a plan that you and your patient can agree on.
- Help the patient implement the agreed-on plan.

Once you've come up with a diagnosis, you have to determine a treatment plan based on that diagnosis. A treatment plan is something you should arrive at with your patient, rather than handing it to her like a prescription. The more you involve your patient in planning treatment, the more likely that she will follow through with the plan.

Compliance was once a popular term for describing good follow-up, but now that term is being gradually replaced with *adherence*, which implies less passivity. A patient *chooses* to adhere, whereas he is *made* to comply. Researchers have found that when clinicians and patients negotiate a treatment plan together, both adherence and clinical outcomes are improved (Eisenthal et al. 1979). Lazare et al. (1975) have outlined an approach to negotiating a treatment plan that makes good sense, from which the following schema is adapted.

ELICIT THE PATIENT'S AGENDA

Your patient's agenda may not be as obvious as it first appears. You can begin to elicit it with a simple question, such as

> *How do you hope I can help you?*

Note that this is a less confrontational way of asking about your patient's agenda than asking

> *What do you want?*
> *What do you expect?*

At this point, the patient may answer vaguely or put the ball back in your court:

> *I want to feel better.*
> *I don't know. You're the doctor.*

It's often important to clarify what sort of information you're seeking:

> *How were you hoping that I could help you to feel better?*

TIP

Often, patients come into an interview with a few specific requests, such as a desire for medication, therapy, a community referral, a letter to their employer, and so on. Some patients may feel embarrassed about divulging their requests so blatantly and may need some encouragement from you:

> *Sometimes patients have a pretty clear idea of what they'd like, for instance medication, counseling, or a piece of advice about something, a letter to someone. (A normalizing response.)*

However, many patients who come to see a clinician really don't have a specific request or agenda. This is often the case with patients who are new to the mental health care system or who are less familiar with the modern consumer model of health care. Don't force the issue with these patients; if they say that they want to hear what your recommendation is and they'll follow it just because you are the expert, go along with it.

NEGOTIATE A PLAN

Remember that eventual treatment adherence is enhanced when the patient and practitioner agree on the nature of the problem. The next phase of negotiation involves arriving at this agreement. If you and your patient agree at the outset about a plan, go directly to the implementation phase. However, often enough, you'll find that your patient's request is either unrealistic or not clinically indicated. Thank your stars that you elicited the request with time to spare, because now you must negotiate a mutually agreed-on goal. Each negotiation will be different, depending on the nature of the request. Creativity is a plus.

Common problematic requests, along with possible negotiation strategies, are as follows:

Request: Your patient asks you for medication, but you cannot prescribe.

Strategy: Determine how urgent the need for medication is. If it's not urgent, make a referral to a psychiatrist, and teach the patient a psychological method for symptom relief, such as relaxation exercises, hypnosis, or cognitive restructuring. Now is a good time to reach into your file of patient handouts. If the need is urgent, refer the patient to an emergency room or crisis clinic, leaving enough time for you to call the clinic to inform the psychiatrist of the patient's diagnosis and medication needs.

Request: Your patient asks for inappropriate medication, such as benzodiazepines for someone with a history of benzodiazepine abuse or antidepressants for mild or transient depressive symptoms.

Strategy: Present a minilecture about the patient's disorder, complete with handouts and recommendations of books.

Request: The patient seeks hospitalization for a problem that can be treated in an outpatient setting.

Strategy: This has become an increasingly problematic request in our era of managed care, and patients may need some education about this issue:

> *These days, insurance companies rarely pay for hospitalizations unless the patient is suicidal, because we have a lot of outpatient treatments that work well.*

An important thing to keep in mind is the possibility that the patient is suffering much more than she originally indicated and that her request for hospitalization is her way of obliquely disclosing that. You may need to reassess her for SI at this point. If you're still satisfied that hospitalization is not indicated, discuss some other options, such as

Day hospitalization
Respite care
Staying with a friend or relative for a while if the home situation is intolerable

Taking a few days off from work
Having the patient call you (or another clinician) for daily
check-ins during a crisis period
Setting up more frequent appointments
A short course of an antianxiety medication

IMPLEMENTING THE AGREED-ON PLAN

Your agreed-on plan will likely fall into one or both of the
following categories:

- A follow-up therapy appointment with you or someone
  else
- Medication trial

Follow-Up Appointments

Your job is to increase the chances that your patient will
show up at the follow-up appointment, regardless of where
that is. You've already contributed to this cause by involving
the patient in the process of deciding on a plan. What more
can you do?

The research shows that the highest follow-up adherence
rates occurred under the following circumstances (Eisenthal
et al. 1979):

- The wait for follow-up appointments is short.
- Referrals are made to specific clinicians rather than to a
  clinic.
- Specific appointments are made at the time of disposition.
- The patient speaks directly to someone at the referral
  clinic during the evaluation session.

The closer you can come to implementing these guidelines,
the better. Of course, this requires plenty of preinterview
preparation (see Chapter 2 on logistical preparation), including the following:

- Have an efficient system for booking your follow-up
  appointments.
- Have a list of specific clinicians who do not have excessive waiting periods for appointments.
- Have a list of referral clinics with their phone numbers
  so your patient can call and make the appointment from
  your office.

Medication Trials

If you have truly collaborated with your patient in deciding on a medication trial, you're well on your way toward achieving adherence to the regimen. Here are some practical issues regarding medications and suggestions for dealing with them:

1. Determine how your patient will pay for medication. While most insurance companies pay for medications, copays vary widely, depending on what was prescribed and the generosity of the insurance company's benefits. Some patients can't afford the copays, and if so, you may be able to provide samples, depending on their availability at your clinic.
2. Make sure your patient understands the side effect profile of the medication.
3. Simplification increases recall and compliance. Thus, instead of "Take 20 mg of Prozac once a day and 50 mg of trazodone at night, as needed for insomnia," say, "Take the green capsule every morning and the white pill at night if you can't sleep."
4. Having your patient repeat what you say increases her recall of your instructions.

Writing Up the Results of the Interview

I've had a long and stormy relationship with the dreaded write-up. During medical school, the requirement of a novell-length write-up was a welcome reprieve from the stresses of rounding on patients and making oral presentations. In residency, I became annoyed with the write-up, which seemed a pesky intrusion into the limited time I had to spend with patients. At the end of a long day, I would sit down heavily at the Dictaphone (remember those?) and try to gather my thoughts, hoping that the resulting transcription would be coherent.

It wasn't until I had been in clinical practice for a few years that I came to terms with the write-up. Having come full circle, I'm back to (sort of) liking it, viewing it as a welcome few minutes of quiet thought and synthesis between patient appointments.

I hope this chapter helps you to work through some of the more painful moments in your own relationship with the write-up. I outline some formats for you to choose among, and I provide some tips to help you streamline the process.

Every write-up represents a balancing act among three objectives:

1. Thoroughness
2. Time efficiency
3. Readability

The ideal write-up incorporates all three objectives. It is thorough enough to document the basis for a diagnosis and treatment plan; it does not require so much time that it would be unfeasible for a busy clinician to produce; and it is not so lengthy as to provoke sighs from equally busy colleagues who must read the write-up because of their involvement in the patient's treatment.

In general, a write-up should not take you more than 10 to 15 minutes to produce, whether you dictate it or write it yourself. It should not be longer than two or three typed pages if you really want colleagues to read it. If you use electronic health records (EHRs) for documentation, you may be constrained by the particular software you or your employer has chosen. At their worse, EHR write-ups become clicking fests through dozens of checkboxes defining different aspects of the mental status exam. I recommend that you use the free-text fields when possible, so that you can build up a narrative picture of your patient that will be more informative to you and others.

IDENTIFYING DATA

The identifying data should be a fairly long initial sentence that sets the stage for the entire evaluation. You want to not only identify who the patient is but also to locate her within the context of social and cultural norms. This includes age, sex, marital status, and source of referral at a minimum and may include other information such as occupation, living situation, and presence of other family.

This is a 45-year-old, twice-married woman with two grown children, who is an accountant for her husband's carpet cleaning business and who was referred by her primary care doctor because of increasing anxiety and the possibility that she is abusing anxiety and pain medication.

or

This is a 29-year-old, single, white man on psychiatric disability, living in a group home downtown, with a long history of paranoid schizophrenia, who was admitted to the hospital after group home staff members found him in the process of drinking a bottle of methyl alcohol in an apparent suicide attempt.

CHIEF COMPLAINT

The chief complaint should be a verbatim sentence of the patient's, usually in response to your question as to the reason he is seeking help.

> *My wife made me come here. There's nothing wrong with me.*
> *My mother just died. I can't deal with it.*
> *I just figured it was time to see a therapist to work out some issues.*

Each of these statements reflects a different sense of purpose and urgency for treatment, and consequently, this information is helpful in setting the stage for the report to follow.

HISTORY OF PRESENT ILLNESS

In Chapter 14, I describe two different definitions of the history of present illness (HPI), one referring to the history of the illness, which may begin years before the interview (history of syndrome approach), and the other referring more narrowly to events of the past few weeks (history of present crisis approach). Which definition to use is a matter of personal or institutional preference. Following are examples of both approaches.

History of Syndrome

Mr. M has a long history of bipolar disorder, beginning in his junior year of college. He was hospitalized for manic behavior, which included studying for days at a time to the point of exhaustion. In addition, he exhibited grandiose, disorganized behavior when he "occupied" the chancellor's outer office and stated that he was the chancellor of the university. He was started on lithium at that point and did well for several years, until he had a series of hospitalizations in the early 1990s for depression and alcohol use after a divorce from his wife.

His last hospitalization was 2 years ago for depression, and he has done fairly well since then, taking medications (venlafaxine [Effexor] and valproic acid [Depakote]) and going to regular therapy and medication appointments.

History of Present Crisis

Mr. M has a long history of bipolar disorder with several hospitalizations but had been doing fairly well for the past 2 years until about 2 weeks ago, when his girlfriend noticed a pattern of manic behavior, which began after a promotion to a new position at his company. He has slept an average of 3 hours a night because of a need to "prepare for his day," he has been talking more rapidly than usual, and he has been making unrealistic plans to become the president of his company. He consented to this admission on the advice of his girlfriend and his outpatient caregivers.

PAST PSYCHIATRIC HISTORY

The nature of the past psychiatric history (PPH) section of your write-up depends on how thorough you have been in the HPI. Generally, the PPH is a time to go into some detail on what sort of psychiatric treatment your patient has had in the past. In Chapter 15, I recommend the mnemonic Go CHa MP as a way of organizing your questioning, and you can also use this for your write-up. You can begin with a General statement, such as

The patient feels that he has received fairly intense, and overall successful, treatment for his depression over the years.

or

The patient has started treatment at various times but by his own admission has been generally noncompliant.

In CHaMP, the C is for current Caregivers, if any. Documenting Hospitalizations is straightforward, and usually the detail is limited by your patient's memory. Noting the date of the last hospitalization is important, because it has implications for the severity of the current problem. Having a separate heading for "Medication trials" is often very helpful, both for other caregivers and for easy reference if you have to make a medication change several months or years after the first visit. Finally, documentation about past Psychotherapy should include a note about whether the patient found it helpful and why or why not.

SUBSTANCE USE HISTORY

Where in the evaluation should you document history of substance use? This varies by practitioner, with some including it in the PPH, others in the social history, and still others in the medical history, usually under "habits." My preference is to use a main heading devoted to the issue, because it is such an important and often overlooked part of the psychiatric history.

Under substance use, I include tobacco and caffeine use, as well as the usual array of more insidious substances, such as alcohol or cocaine.

REVIEW OF SYMPTOMS

The review of symptoms is where you can really impress your readers with your diagnostic thoroughness. Simply go through the major diagnostic categories, indicating whether the patient met any of the criteria and excluding those that you already mentioned in the HPI and in the substance abuse section, if you have included one.

On review of psychiatric symptoms, the patient denied any history of mania or hypomania. She described a history of frequent panic attacks in the past, with some accompanying agoraphobic avoidance, but said that these events had abated spontaneously 2 years ago. While she considers herself a "perfectionist," she denied frank obsessions or compulsions. There was no history of eating disorders, ADHD, dissociative disorders, or psychotic phenomena. With regard to personality disorders, there was a hint of dependent traits in her description of her relationships with her husband and her best friend.

FAMILY HISTORY

If you draw a genogram directly on the evaluation form, this will suffice for the family psychiatric history, although you may want to add a one-line comment to highlight some facet of the history, such as

The patient has a strong genetic loading for bipolar disorder, as shown in the genogram.

If you are dictating the evaluation, I suggest drawing a genogram on a blank sheet that you can staple to the back of the transcription, with the note "see attached genogram" in the family history section.

SOCIAL HISTORY

The thoroughness and length of the social history depend on clinician preference and the purpose of the evaluation. Obviously, a more lengthy social history is necessary in a psychotherapeutic evaluation than a psychopharmacologic evaluation. In addition, some clinical problems are more influenced by psychosocial issues than others. PTSD, for example, will always require a fairly extensive social history, whereas schizophrenia often develops independently of the social milieu.

At a minimum, your social history should include these pieces of information:

Where your patient was born and raised
Number of siblings
Birth order of patient and siblings
Who was present in the household during the formative years
Educational level
Work history
Marital and parenting history of patient
Typical daily activities other than work

The patient was born and raised in Lowell, Massachusetts, and is the youngest of three children, with a brother aged 50 and a sister aged 53. He describes his childhood as "normal" until his father died in a car accident when the patient was 10 years old, after which his mother was "always depressed." His grades in high school were Bs and Cs, and he went to technical school to study auto mechanics for 2 years. He eventually opened his own auto body business, which he still runs. He married his current wife, Diane, when he was 24, and they now have two children, both girls, ages 21 (Laura) and 24 (Angie). He is close to both of them. He works 6 days a week, and when he is not at work, he often watches television while drinking a beer and occasionally goes fishing with male friends. He described his relationship with his wife with the comment, "We get along."

MEDICAL HISTORY

You may use the mnemonic **MIDAS** to organize the medical history. I usually begin with a statement about the patient's general health, such as:

The patient reports that she is in good overall health.

The patient has suffered a number of chronic medical problems.

List any illnesses, surgeries, prescribed medications, and medication allergies. Note the name of the primary care physician. If you have asked questions from the medical review of systems, note any relevant answers. At a minimum, note whether the patient has had any seizures or head injuries, both of which are often germane to psychiatric problems.

The patient is in good general health and denies any history of major illnesses, surgeries, head injuries, or seizures. She takes no medications aside from birth control pills, and she reports an allergy to penicillin. She has regular gynecologic examinations with Dr. L.

The patient has a significant and complicated medical history, including heart disease, diabetes, and neurologic problems stemming from the diabetes. She had coronary bypass surgery last year. Currently, she has shortness of breath when she walks a half block, and she has constant pain in her feet. She recalls having had a concussion after falling off a horse when she was young, but she denies any seizure history. Her primary care physician is Dr. R, and her medications include insulin, captopril, furosemide (Lasix), potassium supplement, hydrocodone (Vicodin) for pain, and paroxetine (Paxil) (20 mg a day). She once had an allergic reaction to bupropion (Wellbutrin), involving a total body rash.

MENTAL STATUS EXAMINATION

In writing up or dictating the mental status section of your diagnostic evaluation, temporarily shed your clinician's mantle and become a creative writer. Describe your patient so well that a reader would be able to recognize him from your description alone.

Compare the following two descriptions of the same patient:

The patient was a 32-year-old man who was tired but cooperative with the interview. He was disheveled. Eye contact was good. Mood and affect were angry and irritable.

The patient was interviewed in a medical bay of the emergency room. He was lying on his back on a gurney in four-point restraints, wearing a hospital gown. He had received 5 mg of haloperidol (Haldol) intramuscularly shortly before the interview. As I walked in, he lifted his head and looked at me intensely, saying, "Will you get me the hell out of these shackles?" I assured him that I would do so if he posed no danger to himself or others. He was resigned and cooperative from that point on.

The second version gives a more vivid sense of the patient's mental status. Yes, he is angry and irritable, but this is in reaction to something in his environment. Furthermore, he's able to modulate his affect in response to the interviewer's statement, indicating a degree of control over his emotional state not communicated by the first summary. The "disheveled" of the first write-up might imply the self-neglect characteristic of schizophrenia, but in fact it's hard to look anything *but* disheveled when you're in a gurney with your limbs restrained.

That said, professional jargon *does* have its place in the write-up. This is especially true in the description of psychotic thought process (TP) and thought content (TC). Words and phrases such as *tangentiality*, *looseness of associations*, and *ideas of reference* are technical terms with meanings that are understood throughout the mental health field, and they should be used when appropriate. Table 34.1 lists some common jargon-containing statements and some fresher alternatives.

TABLE 34.1. Alternatives to Jargon

Mental Status Jargon	More Descriptive Alternative
She was a cooperative informant.	She answered all questions in full but with a sense of apathy and indifference.
He was well groomed.	He had short brown hair that was washed and combed, and he was clean shaven.
She was disheveled.	She had long black hair that looked stiff and unwashed. Her hands were caked with dirt.
He showed psychomotor retardation; eye contact was poor.	He sat slumped over, was staring at the floor, and was nearly motionless throughout the interview.
Speech was fluent and of low volume.	She spoke in a monotonous and wooden tone, and so softly that I had to lean toward her to understand her words.
Affect was flat and dysthymic.	He appeared sad and morose throughout the interview.

Your MSE can follow the format outlined in Chapter 21 (recall the mnemonic: All Borderline Subjects Are Tough, Troubled Characters). A good strategy is to limit jargon to those aspects of the MSE that are normal and to use more descriptive language for those parts of the examination that are directly relevant to the eventual diagnosis.

This was a well-groomed, pleasant-appearing woman, dressed in a professional suit and smelling strongly of perfume. She presented herself as serious and engaged. Her body was tense; she spoke rapidly and articulately as she related her psychiatric history. She seemed quite anxious, with her hands clenched around her billfold and her feet tapping the floor. Her stated mood was "I'm just barely holding on," and "I'm scared of having a panic attack all the time." Her TP was coherent in content and without hallucinations or delusions, but with some excessive rumination on the theme of getting "just the right medicine." She denied SI. On cognitive screen, concentration and memory were normal.

The patient presented as a somewhat disheveled man with long black hair, scraggly beard, and soiled clothes. He wore horn-rimmed glasses and had the look of an eccentric intellectual. He sat quietly for the most part and volunteered very little information; he seemed apathetic rather than guarded. His affect was bland, with a striking disparity between his stated mood ("I'm headed for a breakdown. I hate this life.") and his affect. His TP was coherent and without any LOA or flight of ideas. TC was impoverished. He denied any current hallucinations but admitted to having heard a voice calling his name "once or twice" over the preceding week. He said he wished he were dead but denied any plan to harm himself. On cognitive screen, concentration and memory were normal.

ASSESSMENT

The assessment should be a brief recapitulation of the overall clinical picture and a discussion of differential diagnosis. Remember that many people who read your write-up will read only this section to get right to the point. Therefore, take pains to make the assessment both concise and informative.

This is a 27-year-old married, white, father of two who presents with a history consistent with bipolar disorder and a current clinical picture of major depression with NVSs of hypersomnia, lethargy, poor concentration, and increased appetite for sweet foods. In addition, he presents with significant anxiety, but he probably does not meet criteria for a discrete anxiety disorder, with the possible exception of GAD. Significant family conflict has contributed to his current illness.

This is a 52-year-old, never-married, African American woman who has a long and complicated history of chronic mental illness, variously diagnosed as schizoaffective disorder and chronic schizophrenia. She presents now in a florid psychotic state with auditory hallucinations, ideas of reference, irritability, anxiety, and lack of sleep for 3 days. The current picture is confusing, and it may represent an irritable manic episode or an agitated depression with psychosis. Medication noncompliance may have been a precipitant, although chronic poverty is a relevant psychosocial factor.

DSM-5 DIAGNOSIS

Earlier versions of DSM included five axes: Axis I, the main psychiatric diagnosis; Axis II, personality disorders and developmental disabilities; Axis III, medical issues; Axis IV, psychosocial issues; and Axis V, global assessment of functioning. DSM-5 dropped this multiaxial system, so now you simply list all the diagnoses, without subcategorizing them.

TREATMENT PLAN

A good, concise treatment plan should include:

- Any diagnostic testing planned (i.e., neuropsychological testing, laboratory tests)
- Plans for medication, if you can prescribe
- Plans for therapy, if needed
- Referrals to other health care practitioners, if applicable
- When you plan to see your patient again

For example:
The plan is to obtain electrolytes, complete blood cell count, and thyroid panel to screen for organic causes of

his symptoms; to start sertraline (Zoloft) at 25 mg per day, increasing to 50 mg per day, as tolerated (patient was informed of, and understood, potential risks and benefits of medication); and to start weekly cognitive behavioral therapy. I will see him again in 1 week.

The plan is to begin psychodynamic therapy to address her grief issues and to refer to a psychiatrist for possible antianxiety medication. I will see her again in 1 week.

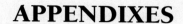

APPENDIXES

Pocket Cards

Psychiatric Evaluation

Section of Evaluation	Relevant Data
Current complaint	
Source	
Identifying data/history of present illness	Chronology, precipitants, neurovegetative symptoms
Past psychiatric history	Go CHaMP
Suicidal ideation/suicide attempt	
Substances	Drug of choice, first use, last use, longest sobriety, detoxifications, history of seizure, delirium tremens
Legal history	
Psychiatric review of symptoms	Depression, mania, anxiety, psychosis, attention deficit hyperactivity disorder, emotional disorder/ disturbance, borderline, schizoid, antisocial
Past medical history	MIDAS, head trauma, brain studies, review of systems
Social history	Raised, abuse, education, work, relationships
Family history	
Mental status examination	Appearance, behavior, speech, mood, affect, thought process, thought content, cognitive
Physical examination	
Narrative assessment	
DSM-IV-TR axes	
Plan	

DSM-5 Mnemonics

Major depression	**SIGECAPS** (4/8)
Dysthymia	**ACHEWS** (2/6)
Manic episode	**DIGFAST** (3/7)
Schizophrenia	**D**elusions **H**erald **S**chizophrenic's **B**ad **N**ews (2/5)
Substance abuse	**T**empted **W**ith **C**ognac (2/11)
Alcoholism	**CAGE** (2/4)
Panic attack	Heart (3) Breathlessness (5) Fear (5) (4/13)
Obsessive-compulsive disorder	**W**ashing and **S**traightening **M**ake **C**lean **H**ouses (1/5)
Posttraumatic stress disorder	**R**emembers **A**trocious **N**uclear **A**ttacks
Generalized anxiety disorder	**M**acbeth **F**rets **C**onstantly **R**egarding **I**llicit **S**ins (3/6)
Bulimia nervosa	**B**ulimics **O**ver-**C**onsume **P**astries (4/4)
Anorexia nervosa	**W**eight **F**ear **B**others anorexics (3/3)
Dementia	**M**emory **LAPSE** (1/6)
Delirium	**M**edical **FRAT** (5/5)
Attention deficit hyperactivity disorder	**MOAT** (6/9)
Borderline personality disorder	**I DESPAIRR**

Note: The numbers in parentheses reflect the number of criteria required for diagnosis out of the total possible criteria.

Defense Mechanisms

Mature defenses	Suppression
	Altruism
	Sublimation
	Humor
Neurotic defenses	Denial
	Repression
	Reaction formation
	Displacement
	Rationalization
Immature defenses	Passive aggression
	Acting out
	Dissociation
	Projection
	Splitting (idealization/ devaluation)
Psychotic defenses	Denial of external reality
	Distortion of external reality

Appearance Terms

Aspect	Appearance Descriptors
Hair	Bald, thinning, close cropped, short, long, shoulder length, crew cut, straight, curly, wavy, frizzy, braided, pony tail, pigtails, afro, relaxed, dreadlocks, unevenly cut, stiff, greasy, dry, matted
Facial hair	Clean shaven, neatly trimmed beard, long scraggly beard, goatee, unshaven
Face	Attractive, nice looking, pleasant, plain, pale, drawn, mongoloid, ruddy, flushed, bony, thin, broad, moon shaped, red nosed, thickly made-up
Eyes (gaze)	Good, shifty, averted, staring, fixated, dilated, downcast, forceful, intense, aggressive, piercing
Body	Thin, cachectic, lean, frail, underweight, normal build, muscular, husky, stocky, overweight, moderately obese, obese, morbidly obese, short, medium height, tall, tattooed arms
Movements	No abnormal movements, fidgety, bobbing knee, facial tic or twitch, lip smacking, lip puckering, tremulous, jittery, restless, wringing hands, motionless, rigid, limp, stiff, slumped
Clothes	Casually dressed, neat, appropriate, professional, immaculate, fashionable, sloppy, ill fitting, outdated, flamboyant, sexually provocative, soiled, dirty, tight, loose, slogans on clothes

Affect Terms

Affect	Terms
Normal	Appropriate, calm, pleasant, relaxed, normal, friendly, comfortable, unremarkable
Happy	Cheerful, bright, peppy, content, self-satisfied, silly, giggly, grandiose, euphoric, elated, exalted
Sad	Sad, gloomy, sullen, depressed, pessimistic, morose, hopeless, discouraged
Anxious	Anxious, worried, tense, nervous, apprehensive, frightened, terrified, bewildered, paranoid
Angry	Angry, irritable, disdainful, bitter, arrogant, defensive, sarcastic, annoyed, furious, enraged, hostile
Indifferent	Indifferent, shallow, superficial, cool, distant, apathetic, aloof, dull, vacant, affectless, uninterested, cynical

Rapid IQ test, Wilson Rapid Approximate Intelligence Test

Intelligence	Best Effort	IQ
Retarded	2 × 6	<70
Borderline	2 × 24	70–80
Dull normal	2 × 48	80–90
Average	2 × 196	90–110

Data from Wilson, I. C. (1967). Rapid approximate intelligence test. *American Journal of Psychiatry, 123*, 1289–1290.

Heritability and Prevalence of Psychiatric Disorders

DSM-5 Disorder	Lifetime Relative Risk if First-degree Relative has Disorder[a]	Lifetime Prevalence in General Population[b]
Bipolar I–II disorders	25	4
Schizophrenia	19	1
Bulimia nervosa	10	2[c]
Panic disorder	10	5
Alcohol abuse	7	13
Generalized anxiety disorder	6	6
Anorexia nervosa	5	1[c]
Specific phobia	3	12
Social anxiety disorder	3	12
Major depression	3	17
Obsessive-compulsive disorder	?	2[b]
Agoraphobia	3	5

[a]Relative risk figures from Reider, R. O., Kaufmann, C. A., and Knowles, J. A. (1994). Genetics. In R. E. Hales, S. C. Yudofsky, and J. A. Talbott (Eds.), *American Psychiatric Press Textbook of Psychiatry*. Washington, DC: American Psychiatric Press. See text for explanation.

[b]Lifetime prevalence figures from Kessler, R. C., Berglund, P., Demler, O., et al. (2005). Lifetime prevalence and age-of-onset distributions of DSM-IV disorders in the national comorbidity survey replication. *Archives of General Psychiatry, 62,* 593–602.

[c]Data from Hudson, J. L., Hiripi, E., Pope, H. G., et al. (2007). The prevalence and correlates of eating disorders in the National Comorbidity Survey Replication. *Biological Psychiatry, 61,* 348–358.

Common DSM-5 Diagnoses

Diagnosis	ICD-9	ICD-10
Alcohol use disorder (moderate)	305.90	F10.20
Anorexia nervosa (restricting type)	307.1	F50.01
Anxiety disorder (unspecified)	300.00	F41.9
Attention deficit hyperactivity disorder, combined type	314.01	F90.2
Bipolar I disorder, depressed episode	296.52	F31.32
Bipolar I disorder, manic episode	296.42	F31.12
Borderline personality disorder	301.83	F60.3
Bulimia nervosa	307.51	F50.2
Delirium (due to general medical condition)	293.0	F05
Major neurocognitive disorder due to Alzheimer's disease	294.10	F02.80
Persistent depressive disorder (dysthymia)	300.4	F341
Generalized anxiety disorder	300.02	F41.1
Major depression, single episode, moderate	296.22	F32.1
Major depression, recurrent, moderate	296.32	F33.1
Obsessive-compulsive disorder	300.3	F42
Panic disorder	300.01	F41.0
Personality disorder, unspecified	301.9	F60.9
Posttraumatic stress disorder	309.81	F43.10
Schizoaffective disorder, bipolar	295.70	F25.0
Schizoaffective disorder, depressive	295.70	F25.1
Schizophrenia	295.90	F60.1
Social anxiety disorder	300.23	F40.10

Age- and Education-adjusted Norms for the Folstein Mini-Mental State Examination (Mean Scores)

Education	Age (yr)														
Level (yr)	18–24	25–29	30–34	35–39	40–44	45–49	50–54	55–59	60–64	65–69	70–74	75–79	80–84	≥85
0–4	22	25	25	23	23	23	23	22	23	22	22	21	20	19
5–8	27	27	26	26	27	26	27	26	26	26	26	25	24	23
9–12	29	29	29	28	28	28	28	28	28	28	27	27	25	26
College and higher	29	29	29	29	29	29	29	29	29	29	28	28	27	27

Data from Crum, R. M., Anthony, J. C., Bassett, S. S., and Folstein, M. F. (1993). Population-based norms for the Mini-Mental State Examination by age and educational level. *Journal of the American Medical Association, 269*, 2386–2391.

Data Forms for the Interview

INITIAL PSYCHIATRIC EVALUATION (SHORT FORM)

Name: _____ Unit number: _____

Date: _____ Date of birth: _____

Insurance: _____

Contacts: _____

Current complaint/HPI:

Past Psychiatric History	**Past Medical History**
Current treaters:	Current medications:
_____	_____
Hospitalizations:	Illnesses:
_____	_____
Medication trials:	Surgeries:
_____	_____
Psychotherapy:	Allergies:
_____	_____
Suicide attempts:	Review of systems: head injury
_____	_____
History violence/incarceration:	Temporal lobe epilepsy:
_____	_____
Substance abuse:	
_____	

Family History

_____

_____

_____

Social/Developmental History

Psychiatric review of systems

Depression   S I G E C A P S

Mania   D I G F A S T

Anxiety disorder: agoraphobic, panic, obsessive-compulsive disorder, posttraumatic stress disorder, generalized anxiety disorder

Psychosis

Attention-deficit hyperactivity disorder, eating disorders

Personality

Mental Status Examination

A B S A T T C

Physical Examination

_____

_____

_____

_____

_____

Laboratory Tests

_____

_____

_____

_____

_____

INITIAL PSYCHIATRIC EVALUATION (LONG FORM)[1]

Name: _____   Referred by: _____

Date: _____   SSN: _____

Address: _____

Date of birth: _____   Occupation: _____

Phone: _____

Insurance: _____

Identifying Information

_____

_____

Presenting Symptoms

_____

_____

History of Present Illness

_____

_____

Past Psychiatric History

_____

_____

Hospitalizations: _____

Medication trials: _____

Psychotherapy: _____

Suicide attempts/gestures: _____

Legal history: _____

---

[1]Adapted from the evaluation form of Anthony Erdmann, M.D.

Substance Use History

Tobacco: _____

Caffeine: _____

Alcohol

CAGE: _____

Withdrawals: _____

Adverse consequences: _____

Last drink: _____

Marijuana: _____

Cocaine/other stimulants: _____

Opiates: _____

Benzodiazepines: _____

Hallucinogens: _____

Detoxification/rehabilitation: _____

Medical History

Primary care physician: _____

Current medications: _____

Illnesses: _____

Surgeries: _____

Drug allergies: _____

Medical Review of Systems

General: _____

Skin: _____

Head, ears, eyes, nose, and throat: _____

Cardiovascular and respiration: _____

Gastrointestinal: _____

Genitourinary/gynecology: _____

Neurology: _____

Family History (Genogram)

Social History

_____

_____

Psychiatric Review of Symptoms

Depression: _____

Mania: _____

Suicidal ideation: _____

Psychosis/schizophrenia

- Symptoms (2/5, 1 month): ___delusions

  ___hallucinations___disorganized speech

  ___disorganized/catatonic behavior

  ___negative symptoms

- Prodrome/residual (1/2, 6 months):

  ___negative symptoms

  ___two positive symptoms

Anxiety

- GAD (3/6, 6 months):___restless___fatigue

  ___conscious___irritable___muscle tension

  ___insomnia

- Panic (4/13, recurrence + 1 month of worry):

  ___shortness of breath___faint___palpitations

  ___trembling___sweating___choking___nauseous

  ___depersonalization/derealization

  ___numbness/tingling chest pain

  ___fear of dying___fear of losing sanity

  ___chills/hot

- OCD:___obsessions___compulsions

  ___interfere/time conscious

- PTSD (1 month):

  Reexperience (1/5):___memories___dreams

  ___flashbacks___distress/reexposure

  ___physiologic reactivity/reexposure

  Avoidance (3/7):___thoughts/feelings

  ___activities/situations___amnesia___less interest

  ___estrangement___restricted affect

  ___thought of no future

  Arousal (2/5):___sleep___irritability

  ___consciousness___hypervigorous___startle

  Social phobia (3/3):___fear/social___exposure/panic

  ___avoid/social

Cognitive

- Dementia: Memory problems

  Other cognitive problems (1/4):___aphasia

  ___apraxia___agnosia___executive functions

- Delirium (5/5):___disturb consciousness

  ___cognitive change___short onset___fluctuate

  ___medication/substance cause

- Attention-deficit hyperactivity disorder:

  Inattentive (6/9):___details/mistakes___attention

  ___listen___follow through___disorganized

  ___avoid/dislike mental effort___loses things

  ___distract___forgetful

  Hyperactive/impulsive (6/9):___fidgets/squirms

  ___diff/seated___runs/climbs___blurts answers

___on/go/motor___diff/play quietly

___talk excess___interrupts/intrudes___waits turn

Somatoform

- Somatization (3/7, starting before age 30, lasting several years):___shortness of breath___dysmenorrhea

  ___burn sex organs___lump/throat___amnesia

  ___vomiting___pain/extremities

- Anorexia (4/4):___refuse/maintain weight

  ___fear of fat___body distortion___amenorrhea

- Bulimia (5/5): ___binge eating___lack of control

  ___inappropriate weight/loss behavior

  ___>2 times/week for 3 months

  ___self-evaluation of body shape

Mental Status Examination

_____

_____

Neurovegetative Symptoms

_____

_____

Cognitive Examination

- rientation: _____

- Concentration: _____

- Memory tests:

  Three objects immediately

  Three objects at 3 minutes

  General information

    Presidents

    World War II

    Current news

Remote personal

Date of wedding

Name of high school/college

Assessment and Diagnostic Formulation

_____

_____

Axis I: _____

Axis II: _____

Axis III: _____

Axis IV: _____

Axis V: _____

Current GAF:

Past year highest GAF: _____

Past year lowest GAF: _____

Treatment Plan

- Medications: _____
- Therapy: _____
- Follow-up: _____

PATIENT QUESTIONNAIRE[2]

Name: _____   Today's date:_____

Date of birth: _____

Address: _____

Telephone numbers

Home: _____

Work: _____

_____

[2]Adapted from the questionnaire of Edward Messner, M.D.

Occupation: _____

Insurance: _____

What is the main concern that led you to consult me?

_____

_____

When did it begin?

_____

_____

Psychiatric History

Outpatient Treatment

Have you ever had outpatient treatment for a psychiatric disorder? _____

If yes, what was the disorder? _____

_____

_____

When and where did you receive treatment? _____

_____

_____

What type of treatment was it (e.g., psychotherapy, medication, behavior therapy, others)? _____

_____

_____

_____

What was the name of your therapist? _____

    Address: _____

    Phone: _____

Do you authorize me to communicate with your therapist?

_____

Hospitalizations

Have you ever been hospitalized for a psychiatric disorder?

_____

If yes, what was the disorder, which hospital(s), and what were the dates? _____

_____

Medication History

What medications are you taking now (medical or psychiatric)?

Drug Dose   Frequency   Prescribing physician

_____

_____

_____

_____

_____

What medications have you taken in the past?

Drug Date Reason for discontinuing

_____

_____

_____

_____

_____

Do you use nonprescription medications?

_____

If yes, which ones? _____

_____

_____

_____

Do you or have you used recreational or illegal drugs?

_____

If yes, which drugs and how much?

_____

_____

Do you drink alcohol? _____

Are you concerned about how much you drink? _____

Are you annoyed at comments about your
drinking? _____

Have you felt guilty about anything resulting from your
drinking? _____

Do you ever have a drink early in the day to calm your
nerves or get rid of a hangover? _____

Do you smoke?_____ If yes, what and how much? _____

Beverages with caffeine:

Coffee_____ Tea_____ Cups per day_____

Colas_____ Others_____ Cans per day_____

Medical History

What illnesses or surgeries have you had in the past?

_____

_____

_____

_____

_____

_____

Do you have any illnesses at present? _____

If yes, please list:

_____

_____

_____

_____

_____

Have you ever had a head injury? _____

When? _____

How did it occur? _____

Have you ever had an EEC or a CT scan of your head?

_____

If yes, when, and what were the results?

_____

_____

Name of your primary care physician: _____

  Address: _____

  Phone: _____

Do you authorize me to communicate with your
physician? _____

Brief Review of Symptoms

Symptoms or problem	No	Yes	Date began	Description
Frequent or severe headaches				
Dizziness/vertigo				
Convulsions or seizures				
Vision problems				
Hearing problems				
Smelling or taste problems				
Thyroid problems				
Cough/asthma				
Chest pain				
Shortness of breath				
Nausea/vomiting/ diarrhea				
Abdominal pain				
Constipation				
Urinary problems				
Arthritis				
Diabetes				
Walking problems				

Social History

Marital status: single_____ married _____ widowed _____ divorced _____

If married, date of wedding: _____

Spouse's date of birth: _____

Spouse's occupation: _____

If widowed, date and cause of spouse's death: _____

_____

If divorced, date and reason for divorce: _____

_____

Children

Name   **Age**   **Location**

_____

_____

_____

_____

Others currently living in your household and their relationship to you:

Name   **Relationship**

_____

_____

_____

_____

Family Medical History

Mother's name: _____

Age: _____ If deceased, date and cause of death: _____

Does (or did) she have any illnesses? _____

Father's name:

Age: _____ If deceased, date and cause of death: _____

Does (or did) he have any illnesses?

_____

Brothers and sisters:

Name   Age   Illnesses

_____

_____

_____

_____

Family Psychiatric History

Has anyone in your family ever had a psychiatric disorder (e.g., depression, mania, schizophrenia, drug or alcohol abuse, anxiety problems, suicide attempts)? _____

If yes, please indicate nature of problem and the family member's relationship to you:

_____

_____

_____

_____

Have you ever been exposed to abuse? _____

 If yes, was it physical?_____ sexual?_____
   emotional?_____

 Who was involved? _____

Educational History

	Name of school	Location	Dates
High school:	_____		
College:	_____		
Postgraduate:	_____		

Occupational History

Dates   Job titles   Reason job ended (if applicable)

_____

_____

_____

_____

_____

_____

Military service:

_____

_____

Adaptive History

What stresses have you overcome in the past?

_____

_____

_____

How did you do it?

_____

_____

What was the best period of your life?

_____

_____

What are your personal strengths?

_____

_____

Patient's signature:

_____

Patient Education Handouts

MAJOR DEPRESSION[1]

Patient Information Handout

Who Gets Depressed?

Major depressive disorder, often referred to as *clinical depression*, is a common illness that can affect anyone. Each year, about 6.7% of US adults experience major depressive disorder. Women are 70% more likely than men to experience depression during their lifetime.

What Is Depression?

Depression is not just "feeling blue" or being "down in the dumps." It is more than being sad or feeling grief after a loss. Depression is an illness (in the same way that diabetes, high blood pressure, and heart disease are illnesses) that affects your thoughts, feelings, physical health, and behaviors day after day.

Depression may be caused by many things, including the following:

- Stressful or depressing life events
- Family history and genetics
- Certain medical illnesses
- Certain medicines
- Drugs or alcohol
- Other psychiatric conditions

Certain life conditions (e.g., extreme stress or grief) may bring on a depression or prevent a full recovery. In some people, depression occurs even when life is going well. Depression is not your fault, nor is it a weakness. It is an illness, and it is treatable.

---

[1]This handout was adapted from public domain information supplied by both the National Institute of Mental Health and the Agency for Health Care Policy and Research (an agency of the U.S. Public Health Service).

How Will I Know Whether I Am Depressed?

People who have major depressive disorder have a number of symptoms nearly every day, all day, for at least 2 weeks. These always include at least one of the following:

- Loss of interest in things you used to enjoy
- Feeling sad, blue, or down in the dumps

You may also have at least three of the following symptoms:

- Feeling slowed down or restless and unable to sit still
- Feeling worthless or guilty
- Increase or decrease in appetite or weight
- Thoughts of death or suicide
- Problems concentrating, thinking, remembering, or making decisions
- Trouble sleeping or sleeping too much
- Loss of energy or feeling tired all of the time

With depression, other physical or psychological symptoms are often present, including the following:

- Headaches
- Other aches and pains
- Digestive problems
- Sexual problems
- Feeling pessimistic or hopeless
- Being anxious or worried

How Is Depression Treated?

Depression is treated with either psychotherapy (counseling) or medications, or with both treatments combined.

Psychotherapy

The most effective psychotherapies for depression are

- Cognitive therapy, in which the therapist points out ways that your thinking is negative and may actually cause you to be more depressed.
- Interpersonal therapy, in which the focus is on improving the quality of your relationships with important people in your life.

Psychotherapy may take one to several months to cure your depression.

Medications

Many effective medications for depression exist. The most commonly prescribed are the selective serotonin reuptake inhibitors (SSRIs), which have names like Prozac, Zoloft, Celexa, and others. Other popular antidepressants include Effexor, Cymbalta, and Wellbutrin. These newer medications have fewer side effects when compared with older medications, such as the tricyclics and the MAOIs.

When someone begins taking an antidepressant, improvement generally will not begin to show immediately. With most of these medications, it will take from 1 to 3 weeks before changes begin to occur. Some symptoms diminish early in treatment; others, later. For instance, a person's energy level or his sleeping or eating patterns may improve before his depressed mood lifts. If there is little or no change in symptoms after 5 to 6 weeks, a different medication may be tried. Some people will respond better to one than to another. Because there is no way of determining beforehand which medication will be effective, the doctor may have to prescribe first one, then another, until an effective medication is found. Treatment is continued for a minimum of several months and may last up to a year or more.

BIPOLAR DISORDER[2]

Patient Information Handout

What Is Bipolar Disorder?

Bipolar disorder, which is also known as *manic-depressive illness*, is a mental illness involving episodes of serious mania and depression. The person's mood usually swings from overly high and irritable to sad and hopeless and then back again, with periods of normal mood in between. Bipolar disorder typically begins in adolescence or early adulthood and continues throughout life. At least two million Americans suffer from manic-depressive illness. Bipolar disorder tends to run in families and is believed to be inherited in many cases.

Key Features of Bipolar Disorder

Bipolar disorder involves cycles of mania and depression.

Signs and symptoms of **mania** *include discrete periods of*

- Increased energy, activity, restlessness, racing thoughts, and rapid talking
- Excessive high or euphoric feelings
- Extreme irritability and distractibility
- Decreased need for sleep
- Unrealistic beliefs in one's abilities and powers
- Uncharacteristically poor judgment
- A sustained period of behavior that is different from usual
- Increased sexual drive
- Abuse of drugs, particularly cocaine, alcohol, and sleeping medications
- Provocative, intrusive, or aggressive behavior
- Denial that anything is wrong

---

[2]This handout was adapted from public domain information supplied by the National Institute of Mental Health.

Signs and symptoms of **depression** include discrete periods of

- Persistent sad, anxious, or empty mood
- Feelings of hopelessness or pessimism
- Feelings of guilt, worthlessness, or helplessness
- Loss of interest or pleasure in ordinary activities, including sex
- Decreased energy, a feeling of fatigue or of being "slowed down"
- Difficulty concentrating, remembering, or making decisions
- Restlessness or irritability
- Sleep disturbances
- Loss of appetite and weight or weight gain
- Chronic pain or other persistent bodily symptoms that are not caused by physical disease
- Thoughts of death or suicide; suicide attempts

How Is Bipolar Disorder Treated?

The most effective treatment for bipolar disorder is one of a variety of mood-stabilizing medications. The most well known of these is **lithium**, which was the first medication introduced for bipolar disorder. Other mood stabilizers include **Tegretol** and **Depakote**. In addition, there are many antipsychotics that are also effective for bipolar disorder. Although all medications for bipolar disorder are effective, side effects, including sedation, weight gain, and light-headedness, often occur. Psychiatrists can minimize these side effects by adjusting the dosage and formulation of medications.

In addition to medications, psychotherapy is helpful, especially during the depressed phase of bipolar disorder. Combination treatment (medications in combination with therapy) leads to the best results for most patients.

PANIC DISORDER[3]

Patient Information Handout

- "It started 10 years ago. I was sitting in a seminar in a hotel and this thing came out of the clear blue. I felt like I was dying."
- "For me, a panic attack is almost a violent experience. I feel like I'm going insane. It makes me feel like I'm losing control in a very extreme way. My heart pounds really hard, things seem unreal, and there's this very strong feeling of impending doom."
- "Between attacks there is this dread and anxiety that it's going to happen again. It can be very debilitating, trying to escape those feelings of panic."

What Is Panic Disorder?

People with panic disorder have feelings of terror that strike suddenly and repeatedly with no warning. They can't predict when an attack will occur, and many develop intense anxiety between episodes, worrying when and where the next one will strike. Between episodes, they feel a persistent, lingering worry that another attack could come any minute. When a panic attack strikes, your heart most likely pounds, and you may feel sweaty, weak, faint, or dizzy. Your hands may tingle or feel numb, and you might feel flushed or chilled. You may have chest pain or smothering sensations, a sense of unreality, or fear of impending doom or loss of control. You may genuinely believe you're having a heart attack or stroke, losing your mind, or on the verge of death. Attacks can occur any time, even during nondream sleep. Most attacks average a couple of minutes, but occasionally, they can go on for up to 10 minutes. In rare cases, they may last an hour or more.

Panic disorder is often accompanied by other conditions, such as depression or alcoholism, and may spawn phobias, which can develop in places or situations where panic attacks have occurred. For example, if a panic attack strikes while

---

[3]This handout was adapted from public domain information supplied by both the National Institutes of Health and the National Institute of Mental Health.

you're riding an elevator, you may develop a fear of elevators and start avoiding them. Some people's lives become greatly restricted—they avoid normal, everyday activities such as grocery shopping, driving, or even leaving the house. They may be able to confront a feared situation only if accompanied by a spouse or other trusted person. Basically, they avoid any situation they fear would make them feel helpless if a panic attack occurred. When people's lives become so restricted by the disorder, as happens in about one third of all people with panic disorder, the condition is called *agoraphobia*. A tendency toward panic disorder and agoraphobia runs in families. Nevertheless, early treatment of panic disorder can often stop the progression to agoraphobia.

Panic attack symptoms include

- Pounding heart
- Chest pains
- Light-headedness or dizziness
- Nausea or stomach problems
- Flushes or chills
- Shortness of breath or a feeling of smothering or choking
- Tingling or numbness
- Shaking or trembling
- Feelings of unreality
- Terror
- A feeling of being out of control or going crazy
- Fear of dying
- Sweating

Who Gets Panic Disorder?

Panic disorder strikes at least 1.6% of the population and is twice as common in women as in men. It can appear at any age, but most often it begins in young adults. Not everyone who experiences panic attacks will develop panic disorder—for example, many people have one attack but never have another. For those who do have panic disorder, though, it's important to seek treatment.

How Is Panic Disorder Treated?

Studies have shown that proper treatment—a type of psychotherapy called *cognitive-behavioral therapy*, medications, or possibly a combination of the two—helps 70% to 90%

of people with panic disorder. Significant improvement is usually seen within 6 to 8 weeks. Cognitive-behavioral approaches teach patients how to view the panic situations differently and demonstrate ways to reduce anxiety (e.g., using breathing exercises or techniques to refocus attention). *Exposure therapy*, a technique used in cognitive-behavioral therapy, often helps to alleviate the phobias that may result from panic disorder. In exposure therapy, people are very slowly exposed to the fearful situation until they become desensitized to it. Some people find the greatest relief from panic disorder symptoms when they take certain prescription medications. Such medications, like cognitive-behavioral therapy, can help to prevent panic attacks or reduce their frequency and severity. Two types of medications that have been shown to be safe and effective in the treatment of panic disorder are antidepressants and benzodiazepines.

OBSESSIVE-COMPULSIVE DISORDER[4]

Patient Information Handout

What Is Obsessive-Compulsive Disorder?

Obsessive-compulsive disorder (OCD), one of the anxiety disorders, is a potentially disabling condition that can persist throughout a person's life. The individual who suffers from OCD becomes trapped in a pattern of repetitive thoughts and behaviors that are senseless and distressing but extremely difficult to overcome. OCD occurs in a spectrum from mild to severe; if severe and untreated, it can destroy a person's capacity to function at work, school, or even home.

How Common Is Obsessive-Compulsive Disorder?

For many years, mental health professionals thought of OCD as a rare disease, because only a minority of their patients had the condition. The disorder often went unrecognized because many of those afflicted with OCD, in efforts to keep their repetitive thoughts and behaviors secret, failed to seek treatment. However, a survey conducted in the early 1980s by the National Institute of Mental Health showed that OCD affects more than 2% of the population, making it more common than such severe mental illnesses as schizophrenia, bipolar disorder, or panic disorder. OCD strikes people of all ethnic groups. Men and women are equally affected.

Key Features of Obsessive-Compulsive Disorder
Obsessions

Obsessions are unwanted ideas or impulses that repeatedly well up in the mind of the person with OCD. Common are persistent fears that harm may come to self or a loved one, an unreasonable concern with becoming contaminated, or an excessive need to do things correctly or perfectly. Again and

---

[4]This handout was adapted from public domain information supplied by the National Institute of Mental Health.

again, the individual experiences a disturbing thought, such as, "My hands may be contaminated—I must wash them," "I may have left the gas on," or "I am going to injure my child." These thoughts are intrusive, unpleasant, and produce a high degree of anxiety. Sometimes, the obsessions are of a violent or a sexual nature, or they concern illness.

Compulsions

In response to their obsessions, most people with OCD resort to repetitive behaviors called *compulsions*. The most common of these are washing and checking. Other compulsive behaviors include counting (often while performing another compulsive action such as hand-washing), repeating, hoarding, and endlessly rearranging objects in an effort to keep them in precise alignment. Mental problems, such as mentally repeating phrases, making lists, or checking, are also common. These behaviors generally are intended to ward off harm to self or others. Some people with OCD have regimented rituals; others have rituals that are complex and changing. Performing rituals may give the person with OCD some relief from anxiety, but it is only temporary.

How Is Obsessive-Compulsive Disorder Treated?

OCD is treated with either psychotherapy (counseling) or medications, or with both treatments combined.

Psychotherapy

The most effective psychotherapy for OCD is cognitive-behavioral therapy. In this technique, your therapist will have you practice exposing yourself to those situations that make you anxious and cause you to act out a compulsion (such as checking or washing). Your therapist will help you to prevent the OCD response. Some of the exposure is done in the therapist's office, but most of it is done at home and is assigned as "homework."

Cognitive-behavioral therapy is very effective, especially for those patients who suffer primarily from compulsions. In such patients, therapy is often more effective than medication.

Medications

Many effective medications for OCD exist. The most commonly prescribed are the SSRIs, which have names like Prozac, Zoloft, Paxil, and Luvox. These are popular because they have very few side effects when compared with older medications. Another effective medication is Anafranil, which tends to have more side effects than the SSRIs.

When someone begins taking an OCD medication, improvement generally will not begin to show up immediately. With most of these medications, it takes from 1 to 3 weeks before changes begin to occur. If there is little or no change in symptoms after 5 to 6 weeks, a different medication may be tried. Because there is no way of determining beforehand which medication will be effective, the doctor may have to prescribe first one, then another, until an effective medication is found. Treatment is continued for a minimum of several months and may last up to a year or more.

References

Ainslie, N. K., & Murden, R. A. (1993). Effect of education on the clock-drawing dementia screen in non-demented elderly persons. *Journal of the American Geriatrics Society, 41*(3), 249–252.

American Psychiatric Association. (2013). *Diagnostic and Statistical Manual of Mental Disorders*, 5th ed. Washington, DC: American Psychiatric Association.

Andreasen, N. C. (1979). Thought, language, and communication disorders. I. Clinical assessment, definition of terms, and evaluation of their reliability. *Archives of General Psychiatry, 36*, 1315–1321.

Andreasen, N. C. (1982). Negative symptoms in schizophrenia: Definition and reliability. *Archives of General Psychiatry, 39*, 784–788.

Andreasen, N. J., Tsuang, M. T., and Canter, A. (1974). The significance of thought disorder in diagnostic evaluations. *Comprehensive Psychiatry, 15*, 27–34.

Anthony, J. C., LeResche, L., Niaz, U., et al. (1982). Limits of the 'Mini-Mental State' as a screening test for dementia and delirium among hospital patients. *Psychological Medicine, 12*, 397–408. doi: 10.1017/S0033291700046730.

Asnis, G. M., Kaplan, M. L., van Praag, H. M., et al (1994). Homicidal behaviors among psychiatric outpatients. *Hospital and Community Psychiatry, 45*, 127–132.

Azar, B. (1997). Poor recall mars research and treatment. *The APA Monitor, 28*, 1.

Baekeland, F., and Lundwall, L. (1975). Dropping out of treatment: A critical review. *Psychological Bulletin, 82*, 738–783.

Barlow, D. (Ed.). (2014). *Clinical Handbook of Psychological Disorders*, 5th ed. New York, NY: The Guilford Press.

Barlow, D. H., Gorman, J. M., Shear, M. K., et al. (2000). Cognitive-behavioral therapy, imipramine, or their combination for panic disorder: A randomized controlled trial. *Journal of the American Medical Association, 283*, 2529–2536.

Basco, M. R., Bostic, J. Q., Davies, D., et al. (2000). Methods to improve diagnostic accuracy in a community mental health setting. *American Journal of Psychiatry, 157*, 1599–1605.

Beckman, H. B., and Franckel, R. M. (1984). The effect of physician behavior on the collection of data. *Annals of Internal Medicine, 101*, 692–696.

Biederman, J. (1991). Attention deficit hyperactivity disorder (ADHD). *Annals of Clinical Psychiatry, 3*, 9–22.

Binder, R. L., and McNiel, D. E. (1996). Application of the Tarasoff ruling and its effect on the victim and the therapeutic relationship. *Psychiatric Services*, *47*, 1212–1215.

Blacker, D., and Tsuang, M. T. (1992). Contested boundaries of bipolar disorder and the limits of categorical diagnosis in psychiatry. *American Journal of Psychiatry*, *149*, 1473–1483.

Bradburn, N. M., Sudman, S., and Wansink, B. (2004). *Asking Questions: The Definitive Guide to Questionnaire Design*. San Francisco, CA: Jossey-Bass.

Brown, T. A., Campbell, L. A., Lehman, C. L., et al. (2001). Current and lifetime comorbidity of the DSM-IV anxiety and mood disorders in a large clinical sample. *Journal of Abnormal Psychology*, *110*, 585–599.

Chang, J., and Nylund, D. K. (2013). Narrative and solution-focused therapies: A twenty-year retrospective. *Journal of Systemic Therapies*, *32*(2), 72–88.

Chochinov, H. M., Wilson, K. G., Enns, M., et al. (1997). Are you depressed? Screening for depression in the terminally ill. *American Journal of Psychiatry*, *154*, 674–676.

Cloninger, C. R., Sigvardsson, S., and Bohman, M. (1996). Type I and type II alcoholism: An update. *Alcohol Health & Research World*, *20*, 18–23.

Cox, A., Holbrook, D., and Rutter, M. (1981a). Psychiatric interviewing techniques. VI. Experimental study: Eliciting feelings. *British Journal of Psychiatry*, *139*, 144–152.

Cox, A., Hopkinson, K., and Rutter, M. (1981b). Psychiatric interviewing techniques. II. Naturalistic study: Eliciting factual information. *British Journal of Psychiatry*, *138*, 283–291.

Cox, A., Rutter, M., and Holbrook, D. (1988). Psychiatric interviewing techniques. A second experimental study: Eliciting feelings. *British Journal of Psychiatry*, *152*, 64–72.

Crook, T., Ferris, S., McCarthy, M., et al. (1980). Utility of digit recall tasks for assessing memory in the aged. *Journal of Consulting and Clinical Psychology*, *48*, 228–233.

David, A., and Fleminger, S. (2012). *Lishman's Organic Psychiatry: A Textbook of Neuropsychiatry*. Boston, MA: Wiley-Blackwell.

Eisenthal, S., Emery, R., Lazare, A., et al. (1979). "Adherence" and the negotiated approach to patienthood. *Archives of General Psychiatry*, *36*, 393–398.

Elstein, A. S., Shulman, L. S., and Sprafka, S. A. (1978). *Medical Problem-Solving: An Analysis of Clinical Reasoning*. Cambridge, MA: Harvard University Press.

Ewing, J. A. (1984). Detecting alcoholism. The CAGE questionnaire. *Journal of the American Medical Association*, *252*, 1905–1907.

Felthous, A. R. (1991). Duty to warn or protect: Current status for psychiatrists. *Psychiatric Annals, 21,* 591–598.

First, M. (2013). *DSM-5 Handbook of Differential Diagnosis.* Washington, DC: American Psychiatric Press.

Flaum, M. (1995). The diagnosis of schizophrenia. In C. Shriqui, and H. Nasrallah (Eds.), *Contemporary Issues in the Treatment of Schizophrenia.* Washington, DC: American Psychiatric Press.

Folstein, M. F., Folstein, S. E., and McHugh, P. R. (1975). "Mini-mental state." A practical method for grading the cognitive state of patients for the clinician. *Journal of Psychiatric Research, 12,* 189–198.

Frank, J. D., and Frank, J. B. (1991). *Persuasion and Healing.* Baltimore, MD: The Johns Hopkins University Press.

Frank, E., Kupfer, D. J., and Siegel, L. R. (1995). Alliance not compliance: A philosophy of outpatient care. *Journal of Clinical Psychiatry, 56*(suppl 1), 11–16.

Hall, R. C., Gardner, E. R., Stickney, S. K., et al. (1980). Physical illness manifesting as psychiatric disease. II. Analysis of a state hospital inpatient population. *Archives of General Psychiatry, 37,* 989–995.

Harwood, D. M., Jr., Hope, T., and Jacoby, R. (1997). Cognitive impairment in medical inpatients. I. Screening for dementia—Is history better than mental state? *Age and Ageing, 26,* 31–35.

Havens, L. (1986). *Making Contact.* Cambridge, MA: Harvard University Press.

Hinton, J., and Withers, E. (1971). The usefulness of clinical tests of the sensorium. *British Journal of Psychiatry, 119,* 9–18.

Honig, A., Romme, M. A. J., and Ensink, B. J. (1998). Auditory hallucinations: A comparison between patients and nonpatients. *Journal of Nervous Mental Disorders, 186,* 646–651.

Isaacs, B., and Kennie, A. (1973). The set test as an aid to the detection of dementia in old people. *British Journal of Psychiatry, 123,* 467–470.

Jacobs, M., Frank, E., Kupfer, D. J., et al. (1987). A psychoeducational workshop for depressed patients, family, and friends: Description and evaluation. *Hospital and Community Psychiatry, 38,* 968–972.

Jones, P. B. (2013). Adult mental health disorders and their age at onset. *British Journal of Psychiatry, 202,* s5–s10.

Jorm, A., Scott, R., Cullen, J. S., et al. (1991). Performance of the Informant Questionnaire on Cognitive Decline in the Elderly (IQCODE) as a screening test for dementia. *Psychological Medicine, 21,* 785–790.

Kaplan, C. (2011). Hypothesis testing. In M. J. Lipkin, S. M. Putnam, and A. Lazare (Eds.), *The Medical Interview.* New York, NY: Springer-Verlag.

Keller, M. B., and Manschreck, T. C. (1989). The mental status examination. II. Higher intellectual functioning. In A. Lazare (Ed.), *Outpatient Psychiatry: Diagnosis and Treatment*. Baltimore, MD: Williams & Wilkins.

Kessler, R. C., Berglund, P., Demler, O., et al. (2005). Lifetime prevalence and age-of-onset distributions of DSM-IV disorders in the national comorbidity survey replication. *Archives of General Psychiatry*, *62*, 593–602.

Klein, D. N., Riso, L. P., and Anderson, R. L. (1993). DSM-III-R dysthymia: Antecedents and underlying assumptions. *Progress in Experimental Perspectives in Psychopathologic Research*, *16*, 222–253.

Lam, R. W., and Stewart, J. N. (1996). The validity of atypical depression in DSM-IV. *Comprehensive Psychiatry*, *37*, 375–383.

Lazare, A., Eisenthal, S., and Wasserman, L. (1975). The customer approach to patienthood—Attending to patient requests in a walk-in clinic. *Archives of General Psychiatry*, *32*, 553–558.

Lejoyeux, M., Ades, J., Tassain, V., et al. (1997). Phenomenology and psychopathology of uncontrolled buying. *American Journal of Psychiatry*, *153*, 1524–1529.

Lipkin, M. L. (2002). The medical interview and related skills. In W. T. Branch, Jr. (Ed.), *Office Practice of Medicine*. Philadelphia, PA: W. B. Saunders.

Llark, C. M., Sheppard, L., Fillenbaum, G. G., et al. (1999). Variability in annual Mini-Mental State Examination score in patients with probably Alzheimer disease. *Archives of Neurology*, *56*, 857–862.

Manly J. J., Jacobs D. M., Sano M., et al. (1999). Effect of literacy on neuropsychological test performance in nondemented, education-matched elders. *Journal of the International Neuropsychological Society*, *5*(3), 191–202.

Marshall, P., Schroeder, R., O'Brien, J., et al. (2010). Effectiveness of symptom validity measures in identifying cognitive and behavioral symptom exaggeration in adult attention deficit hyperactivity disorder. *The Clinical Neuropsychologist*, *24*, 1204–1237.

McKenna, P. J. (1994). *Schizophrenia and Related Syndromes*. Oxford, UK: Oxford University Press.

Meagher, J., Leonard, M., Donoghue, L., et al. (2015). Months backward test: A review of its use in clinical studies. *World Journal of Psychiatry*, *22*, 305–314.

Miller, G. A. (1957). The magical number seven, plus or minus: Some limits on our capacity for processing information. *Psychological Review*, *63*, 81–97.

Milstein, V., Small, J. G., and Small, I. F. (1972). The subtraction of serial sevens test in psychiatric patients. *Archives of General Psychiatry*, 26, 439–441.

Morrison, J. (2014). *The First Interview*. New York, NY: The Guilford Press.

Morrison, J., and Munoz, R. A. (2009). *Boarding Time: A Psychiatry Candidate's Guide to Part II of the ABPN Examination*. Washington, DC: American Psychiatric Press.

Mueser, K. T., and Glynn, S. M. (1999). *Behavioral Family Therapy for Psychiatric Disorders*, 2nd ed. Oakland, CA: New Harbinger Publications.

Murden, R. A., McRae, T. D., Kaner, S., et al (1991). Mini-Mental State exam scores vary with education in blacks and whites. *Journal of the American Geriatric Society*, 39, 149–155.

Norton, G. R., Dorward, J., and Cox, B. J. (1986). Factors associated with panic attacks in nonclinical subjects. *Behavior Therapy*, 17, 239–252.

Othmer, E., and Othmer, S. C. (2001). *The Clinical Interview Using DSM-IV-TR*. Washington, DC: American Psychiatric Press.

Patterson, W. M., Dohn, H. H., Bird, J., et al. (1983). Evaluation of suicidal patients: The SAD PERSONS scale. *Psychosomatics*, 24, 343–349.

Payne, S. L. (1951). *The Art of Asking Questions*. Princeton, NJ: Princeton University Press.

Pekarik, G. (1993). Beyond effectiveness: Uses of consumer-oriented criteria in defining treatment success. In T. Giles (Ed.), *Handbook of Effective Psychotherapy*. New York, NY: Plenum Press.

Pilowsky, I., and Boulton, D. M. (1970). Development of a questionnaire-based decision rule for classifying depressed patients. *British Journal of Psychiatry*, 116, 647–650.

Pinkofsky, H. B. (1997). Mnemonics for DSM-IV personality disorders. *Psychiatric Services*, 48, 1197–1198.

Platt, F. W., and McMath, J. C. (1979). Clinical hypocompetence: The interview. *Annals of Internal Medicine*, 91, 898–902.

Posternak, M. A., and Zimmerman, M. (2003). How accurate are patients in reporting their antidepressant treatment history? *Journal of Affective Disorders*, 75, 115–124.

Rapp, M. S. (1979). Re-examination of the clinical mental status examination. *Canadian Journal of Psychiatry*, 24, 773–775.

Regier, D. A., Farmer, M. E., Rae, D. S., et al. (1990). Comorbidity of mental disorders with alcohol and other drug abuse. *Journal of the American Medical Association*, 264, 2511–2518.

Reider, R. O., Kaufmann, C. A., and Knowles, J. A. (1994). Genetics. In R. E. Hales, S. C. Yudofsky, and J. A. Talbott (Eds.),

American Psychiatric Press Textbook of Psychiatry. Washington, DC: American Psychiatric Press.

Rudd, M. D., Berman, A. L., Joiner, T. E., et al. (2006). Warning signs for suicide: Theory, research, and clinical applications. *Suicide and Life-threatening Behavior*, *36*, 255–262.

Sacks, M. H., Carpenter, W. T., Jr., and Strauss, J. S. (1974). Recovery from delusions. Three phases documented by patient's interpretation of research procedures. *Archives of General Psychiatry*, *30*, 117–120.

Shea, S. C. (1998). *Psychiatric Interviewing: The Art of Understanding*. Philadelphia, PA: W. B. Saunders.

Shea, S. C. (2006). *Improving Medication Adherence*. Philadelphia, PA: Lippincott Williams & Wilkins.

Shea, S. C. (2007). Clinical interviewing: Practical tips from master clinicians. *Psychiatric Clinics of North America*, *30*, 219–225.

Shea, S. C. (2011). *The Practical Art of Suicide Assessment*. Stoddard, NH: Mental Health Presses.

Smith, A. (1967). The serial sevens subtraction test. *Archives of Neurology*, *17*, 78–80.

Solomon, S. D., and Davidson, J. R. T. (1997). Trauma: Prevalence, impairment, service use, and cost. *Journal of Clinical Psychiatry*, *58*(suppl 9), 5–11.

Steinweg, D. L., and Worth, H. (1993). Alcoholism: The keys to the CAGE. *The American Journal of Medicine*, *94*, 520–523.

Stunkard, A. J., Fernstrom, M. H., Price, A., et al. (1990). Direction of weight change in recurrent depression. *Archives of General Psychiatry*, *47*, 857–860.

Sullivan, H. S. (1970). *The Psychiatric Interview*. New York, NY: W. W. Norton and Co.

Tangalos, E. G., Smith, G. E., Ivnik, R. J., et al. (1996). The Mini-Mental State Examination in general medical practice: Clinical utility and acceptance. *Mayo Clinic Proceedings*, *71*, 829–837.

Tardiff, K. (1992). The current state of psychiatry in the treatment of violent patients. *Archives of General Psychiatry*, *49*, 493–499.

Tsoi, K. K., Chan, J. Y., Hirai, H. W., et al. (2015). Cognitive tests to detect dementia: A systematic review and meta-analysis. *JAMA Internal Medicine*, *175*, 1450–1458.

Turner, C. F., Ku, L., Sonenstein, F. L., et al. (1996). Impact of audio-CASI on bias in reporting of male–male sexual contacts. In R. B. Warnecke (Ed.), *Health Survey Research Methods*. Hyattsville, MD: National Center for Health Statistics.

Vaillant, G. E. (1988). Defense Mechanisms. In A. M. Nicholi, Jr. (Ed.), *The New Harvard Guide to Psychiatry*. Cambridge, MA: Harvard University Press.

Vaillant, G. E. (1995). *The Natural History of Alcoholism Revisted.* Cambridge, MA: Harvard University Press.

Weissenburger, J., Rush, A. J., Giles, D. E., et al. (1986). Weight change in depression. *Psychiatry Research*, 17, 275–283.

White, M., and Epston, D. (1990). *Narrative Means to Therapeutic Ends.* New York, NY: W.W. Norton & Company.

Wilson, I. C. (1967). Rapid approximate intelligence test. *American Journal of Psychiatry*, 123, 1289–1290.

Winokur, G. (1981). *Depression: The Facts.* Oxford, UK: Oxford University Press.

Index

Notes: Page numbers followed by "f" denote figures. Page numbers followed by "t" denote tables.